ALL YOU NEED TO KNOW ABOUT

Joint Surgery

Preparing for Surgery, Recovery and an Active New Lifestyle

THE ARTHRITIS FOUNDATION THANKS ZIMMER, INC.,
FOR ITS GENEROUS SUPPORT IN DEVELOPING THIS BOOK.

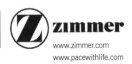

www.zimmer.com
www.pacewithlife.com

ALL YOU NEED TO KNOW ABOUT
Joint Surgery

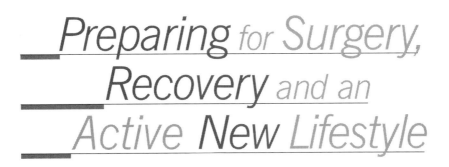

Preparing for Surgery, Recovery and an Active New Lifestyle

By the Arthritis Foundation
Chief Medical Editor: John H. Klippel, MD

AN OFFICIAL PUBLICATION
OF THE ARTHRITIS FOUNDATION

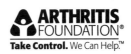

ARTHRITIS FOUNDATION®
Take Control. We Can Help.™

All You Need To Know About Joint Surgery:
Get Ready for Surgery, Recovery and an Active New Lifestyle

By the Arthritis Foundation
Chief Medical Editor: John H. Klippel, MD

An Official Publication of the Arthritis Foundation
Copyright 2002
Arthritis Foundation
1330 West Peachtree Street
Atlanta, GA 30309

Library of Congress Card Catalog Number: 2002106598
ISBN: 0-912423-33-1

Printed in Canada

This book was conceived, designed and produced by the Arthritis Foundation.

The mission of the Arthritis Foundation is to improve lives through leadership
in the prevention, control and cure of arthritis and related diseases.

Editorial Director: Susan Bernstein
Art Director: Susan Siracusa
Interior Illustrations: Kathryn Born
Color Insert Illustrations: Claudia Grosz

 This book was reviewed by members of the
American Academy of Orthopaedic Surgeons.

Table of Contents

Acknowledgements

All You Need To Know About Joint Surgery is a book written for people who are exploring or preparing for joint replacement and other types of joint surgery, as well as for their families and loved ones. While this book should not take the place of the advice and treatment that your physicians and other health-care professionals provide, it may help you better understand your condition and the many treatments available to you at this time.

Special acknowledgements go to the following health-care professionals who donated their time to review this book for medical accuracy: John H. Klippel, MD, Medical Director of the Arthritis Foundation; Patrick Kirk, MD, an orthopaedic surgeon at The University Hospital of Cincinnati and University Orthopaedics and Sports Medicine, Cincinnati; Jeffrey T. Nugent, MD, Clinical Assistant Professor of Orthopaedic Surgery at Emory University and an orthopaedic surgeon at Piedmont Hospital, Atlanta; and Sandy Ganz, PT, a physical therapist working with patients at the Hospital for Special Surgery, New York, NY.

Special acknowledgements should go to Shelly Morrow, who wrote the text of this book. The editorial director of the book is Susan Bernstein. The art director and designer of the cover is Susan Siracusa. Layout production was done by Jill Dible. The medical illustrations were created by Claudia Grosz, and the exercise illustrations were created by Kathryn Born.

This book was made possible through a development grant from Zimmer, Inc., a company that develops, produces and markets orthopaedic products such as joint replacement implants around the world. The Arthritis Foundation would like to thank the American Academy of Orthopaedic Surgeons for their review and assistance.

This book is published by the Arthritis Foundation, the only national, not-for-profit health agency serving the more than 43 million Americans with arthritis or a related disease. The mission of the Arthritis Foundation is to improve lives through leadership in the prevention, control and cure of arthritis and related diseases. This book is inspired by that mission. We hope that its readers will find useful guidance as they explore surgery.

Foreword

Although many people with arthritis will not need to have surgery, for those who do need it, the improvements in quality of life following surgery can be dramatic – in fact, truly a godsend.

After surgery, chronic, often excruciating joint pain is relieved. And, most importantly, surgery can restore joint function, letting people once again fully use their joints to go about their daily lives. Common activities that were once impossible to perform become doable again.

There are many different types of joint surgery available now, some using new, improved technology. Recent advances in total joint replacement of the hip and knee, in particular, have been truly remarkable. Joint replacements are now performed on thousands of people with osteoarthritis, rheumatoid arthritis and other forms of arthritis affecting the lower extremities each day in this country. For these people, surgery allows them to once again walk free of pain.

Joint surgery, however, is only one of many options for people affected by arthritis or related joint diseases. Self-care measures including exercise, diet and lifestyle changes all play an important role in the management of arthritis, along with drugs (including newly developed, powerfully effective medications), physical therapy, and complementary and alternative treatments. For most people with arthritis, some or all of these therapies become part of an overall treatment plan. *All You Need To Know About Joint Surgery* allows you to better understand your numerous treatment options. This knowledge will help you more effectively communicate and work with your physician and other members of your health-care team, so you can develop a treatment plan that works for you.

If you and your physician decide that joint surgery is the best option for your arthritis, inevitably you will have hundreds of questions about what happens before, during and after surgery. Joint surgery is a major undertaking. Making certain that every patient who is considering surgery understands and gets clear answers to their questions before surgery is extremely important. *All You Need To Know About Joint Surgery* provides answers to the most commonly asked questions to help better prepare people for joint surgery and rehabilitation.

The mission of the Arthritis Foundation is to improve lives through leadership in the prevention, control and cure of arthritis and related diseases. The Arthritis Foundation believes that knowledge is power and that the actions taken by people with arthritis play a large and important role in determining their outcome. This book, *All You Need To Know About Joint Surgery*, is a practical and clear guide that will help you better understand the important role of surgery in the treatment of arthritis.

John H. Klippel, MD
Medical Director
Arthritis Foundation

Introduction

When arthritis causes terrible pain in your joints – your knees, your hips, your shoulders, your hands – just walking to your mailbox or doing the dishes seem like overwhelming tasks. When your pain is that severe, you will consider any treatment to make the pain go away. Now more than ever, Americans are turning to surgery, particularly total joint replacement surgery, to address the excruciating pain and life-changing immobility that may result from joint deterioration and damage.

Thankfully, there are many options for treating your pain and the problems caused by arthritis. You and your doctor will likely explore many non-surgical treatments, including drugs, exercise therapy, weight loss, water therapy and more, before you consider having surgery. Surgery, no matter how common the procedure may be, is a major undertaking. You will want to explore many other, non-invasive options for treating your arthritis before you turn to surgery.

But, when you experience pain in your joints that drugs, exercise or other therapies don't treat sufficiently, surgery is the next step to consider. With new advances in joint surgery techniques and development of **prostheses** (the actual joint replacement parts), surgery is now one of the most successful, common treatments for advanced joint pain and immobility.

How – and when – do you decide if joint surgery is right for you? How will you find the right doctor, prepare for surgery and recovery, and talk to your family and employers about your need to have surgery on your joints?

Each year, hundreds of thousands of people in the United States and throughout the world are choosing joint surgery, whether total joint replacement or other types of procedures, as a viable option for reducing pain, restoring mobility and improving quality of life. That's why the Arthritis Foundation has created this book, *All You Need To Know About Joint Surgery* – to inform you about the options you have for surgically replacing or repairing the structures of a painful joint.

No matter what type of surgery you are having, it's important to be fully prepared for the procedure and your recovery. Surgery is a serious endeavor, but this book offers realistic guidance and helpful advice for being as prepared as possible for your operation and recovery. The book will help you prepare yourself physically, emotionally and financially for surgery; offer guidance on how to choose the surgeon that's right for you and to create a positive dialogue with your doctor; prepare your home for the first, delicate days of your recovery; and understand what recovery from joint surgery is really like. We'll explore the various types of surgical procedures being performed on joints today, and we'll try to answer the many questions you may have about joint surgery.

While there are many different types of surgery used to correct various joint disorders, the most common of these procedures is **total joint replacement**. This term refers to knee, hip, shoulder, elbow and other replacements. It's likely that someone you know has had one of these operations, and that you are considering having a joint replacement at some point in the future also. Because this procedure is so common and becoming more so, we will place most of our discussion on that type of surgery in this book. But we will also discuss many other types of surgery performed on joints that correct various serious problems.

If you have arthritis or some type of joint problem or pain that may require surgery, or if you are caring for someone facing joint surgery, *All You Need To Know About Joint Surgery* has a wealth of information to get your life, home, job, mind and body in order before you go into the operating room – so you will be in the best shape to recover from your surgery successfully and get on with an active, fulfilling life!

The Arthritis Foundation is here to help you take control of your arthritis, joint pain and other problems. The chapter nearest you has many resources, including free pamphlets and physician referral services, on hundreds of diseases and problems affecting the joints. Call **800/283-7800** or go to the Arthritis Foundation Web site at **www.arthritis.org** to find the chapter or branch office serving your area and to get helpful information on controlling your pain and increasing your quality of life. At the end of this book, we have included a resources section which explains the many programs, services and information sources the Arthritis Foundation offers to help you take control of your health and lead an active, more fulfilling life.

Now, let's begin our look at joint surgery by discussing the problems that may lead to joint surgery, if you are a candidate for one of these surgeries, and what these procedures might do to reduce your pain and improve your quality of life.

chapter 1:

Do You Need Joint Surgery?

If you have picked up this book, it's probably for one of the follow-ing reasons:

- You have arthritis with severe pain that is limiting your ability to use your joints.
- Your doctor has brought up joint surgery (such as a knee or hip replacement) as an option for relieving that pain.
- Your friends have had or are talking about having joint replacements or other types of joint surgery.
- You have noticed some pain or movement problems in your joints now, and you think you'll face surgery to correct these problems somewhere down the road.

Sound familiar? Joint surgery is a very common procedure today, and these surgeries are increasingly popular treatment options for people with severe pain, swelling and mobility problems in their major joints. There are several reasons why a person might consider joint surgery, and why they might choose to undergo this major medical procedure and lengthy, often tedious recovery program. The main reason is pain. If you are in so much pain that you can't stand it anymore, and if you can't do the everyday things you need and love to do, then surgery doesn't seem so bad.

Nevertheless, the decision to have surgery is a major one. Most people don't relish the thought of undergoing an operation, spending time in the hospital and in recovery if they don't need to. Chances are, if you're reading this, your pain is bad enough – or you think it will be at some point – that you're willing to think about surgery as a treatment.

How Do You Know When It's Time To Consider Surgery?

For each person, the decision to consider surgery is very personal one, and this decision depends on their unique physical, emotional and financial situation. When you decide to explore surgery really depends on your feelings, and how much your pain or other symptoms are affecting your lifestyle and happiness. How will you know when it is time to have joint surgery? As they say about meeting the person you will fall in love with: You'll just know!

The factors on which you base your decision to have surgery will come from a few different sources. One will be your doctor, who can note changes and damage in your joint as well as changes in your ability to move and use your joint. The most important indicator of your need to consider surgery, however, will be yourself and how you feel performing ordinary activities and functions.

Perhaps a joint, such as your knee or shoulder, has bothered you with twinges of pain or stiffness off and on for years. Or maybe the pain and stiffness have occurred regularly, but you've been able to ease those symptoms with over-the-counter pain medication, or topical creams. But over the years, your pain has increased. Maybe you've even had trouble moving the joint well at all. You may be taking pain relievers frequently just to help you get through your day. You may continue to need more and more medicine without getting complete relief.

Your joint may ache so much and be so difficult to move that you may have given up some of your favorite activities, such as sewing, playing tennis or just taking walks around the block. You may even be having trouble at work because the pain or stiffness is so bad. The pain and discomfort may keep you awake at night and prevent you from getting a good night's sleep. Even simple tasks like fixing meals, showering and getting dressed may be very difficult and painful for you.

Perhaps you've even seen your doctor for other solutions and stronger painkilling or inflammation-reducing medications. You may feel frustrated that you've tried so many remedies, yet you don't feel any better and your joint may even be feeling worse.

You may experience one or several of the situations mentioned above that may lead you to start thinking about surgery. The point that links all of these different situations together is the fact that nothing – medications, exercise, alternative therapies, hot and cold packs – has provided adequate pain relief. The problem in your joint begins to affect every part of your life so that you can no longer live the comfortable and active life that you may have been used to.

One of the most common causes of joint pain, and one of the main reasons for surgery, is a condition called **arthritis**. This term literally means joint inflammation. Arthritis often is used to refer to any of the more than 100 musculoskeletal (having to do with the muscles and bones) conditions that affect the joints. The most common type of arthritis is **osteoarthritis**, which currently affects 21 million Americans.

A **joint** is the place where two bones meet and join together, such as the knee, elbow, shoulder, hip, wrist or knuckle. Arthritis affects the structures that make up a joint, causing them to become inflamed or damaged. This damage and inflammation may lead to pain, stiffness and difficulty moving the joint.

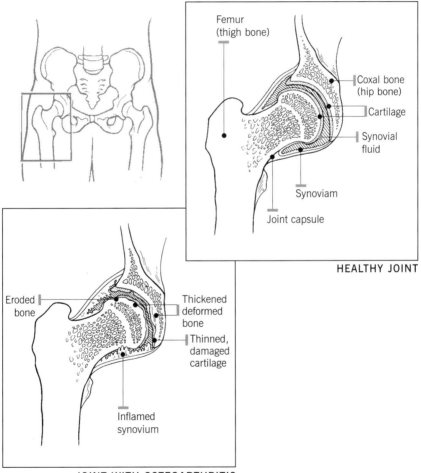

Femur
(thigh bone)

Coxal bone
(hip bone)

Cartilage

Synovial
fluid

Synoviam

Joint capsule

HEALTHY JOINT

Eroded
bone

Thickened
deformed
bone

Thinned,
damaged
cartilage

Inflamed
synovium

JOINT WITH OSTEOARTHRITIS

Having a condition like arthritis is frustrating. You may have to take medication, you have pain, and you may have trouble continuing activities that you once enjoyed. You learn to live with these challenges that come with arthritis. And often, therapies such as drugs, exercise, and heat and cold therapy provide enough relief to help you manage them.

But certain types of arthritis may also be **progressive** diseases. This term means that the joint damage and **inflammation** (swelling) can get worse over time. As this happens, you may have trouble getting the relief you need from your medications and other therapies. There may come a time when the pain and stiffness you face make it difficult for you to perform daily activities, such as bathing yourself, dressing, climbing stairs and even walking comfortably.

You may be relying more on family members and friends to help you do the things you used to handle on your own. Certain tasks at work may be more cumbersome and difficult, causing you to feel more stress and fatigue as well. At this point, surgery may be an option you want to consider in order to reduce pain and improve your ability to function.

You may need to consider joint surgery when:

- You have increased pain that is not helped by drugs or other methods of pain relief.
- Your ability to move comfortably decreases significantly so that you have trouble with daily tasks such as walking, bathing and dressing.
- Your independence is reduced because you need help from friends and family members to take care of yourself.

If you find that these statements are true for you, you may want to start talking with your doctor about joint surgery. Perhaps your doctor has mentioned joint surgery to you before as an option for the future, or maybe he has never discussed it with you.

Joint surgery is a treatment that seeks to relieve pain and improve the mobility of a painful or damaged joint. Surgery can include a number of types of operations, from less invasive to more invasive techniques. These techniques involve removing damaged portions of the joint and sometimes reshaping or replacing parts of the joint.

Perhaps you have friends or relatives who have had total joint replacement surgery. This is just one type of joint surgery that involves completely replacing the painful, damaged joint with metal and plastic joint components. Joint replacement is a very common type of surgery. Each year, more than 260,000 knee replacements and about 160,000 hip replacement operations are performed in the United States. **Arthroscopy** is another common type of joint surgery that you may be familiar with. About 1.5 million arthroscopic knee surgeries are performed each year.

If you do have severe or long-lasting pain or disability in one or more of your joints, it is very important that you see your doctor. Set up an appointment with your primary-care doctor, orthopaedist or other specialist to talk over your many treatment options. He or she may refer you to a surgeon for specific treatments, which we will discuss more later in this book.

What To Ask Your Doctor

If you think you have arthritis, if you have been diagnosed with arthritis in the past and now the pain in one or more of your joints has grown unbearable, or if you have had an injury that may have caused some damage in one of your joints and causes you pain, it's time to make an appointment with your doctor to discuss your options, which may include surgery. Perhaps you have been trying various treatments for arthritis pain for some time, and now you feel that it's time to explore surgery as a treatment option. Your doctor is the place to start.

This appointment may be with your regular **primary-care physician** (such as an internist) or family doctor, or you may choose to make an appointment with a specialist such as an **orthopaedist**. We will discuss these different types of doctors on page 33. But when you make an appointment with a doctor, what should you bring up? It's important to be prepared for this discussion.

Mention changes you have noticed in your pain level recently, or if the pain has lasted for a long time. Try to describe the pain as clearly and specifically as you can. Talk about where it occurs, what it feels like, what motions seem to trigger the pain, etc. Discuss your ability to get around and perform daily tasks. In the days leading up to your appointment, you might take some notes (or keep a health diary, which we will also discuss later) about your problems and the changes you have noticed. Make note of such things as what time of day the pain is at its worst, or if certain activities aggravate your pain.

Jot down what over-the-counter treatments or home remedies you have tried, what seems to work and what seems to do nothing to ease your pain. It's important that you always tell your doctor what medications or dietary supplements you are taking. Write these down so you won't forget! Certain medications can interact with other treatments your doctor might prescribe for you.

Important Items To Discuss With Your Doctor

To prepare for your initial appointment with your doctor to discuss surgery, make notes about the following:

- Recent changes you have noticed in your pain or mobility
- How long the pain in your joint or joints has lasted
- Specific description of the pain
- What motions or activities seem to trigger or worsen the pain
- What time of day the pain is at its worst
- Prescription or over-the-counter treatments you have used or are using
- Alternative or complementary treatments you have used or are using

SAMPLE QUESTIONS FOR YOUR DOCTOR

Your doctor may only be able to spend a limited amount of time with you to discuss your problems and possible treatment steps. So it's important to make the most of that time. Be prepared before you go to the doctor. Spend the time you have with your doctor asking specific questions about joint surgery. If you are seeing a doctor for the first time, make sure you have your medical history (details of any past or current medical problems, drug allergies, past surgeries or medical procedures, chronic illnesses) or any records from your primary-care doctor. Bring a list of questions you may have about surgery, such as these common sample questions:

- What makes someone a good candidate for joint surgery?
- What are the risks involved in joint surgery?
- Would there be any other non-surgical treatments I haven't yet tried that would ease my pain and help me move more easily?
- How would surgery help my particular problem?
- What would not change after the operation?
- How long is the recovery process?
- What is involved in the recovery process?

We will further discuss all of these issues, including even more questions to ask your doctor, in following chapters of this book. When your doctor answers these and other questions you may have, write down the information he or she provides. Preparing for surgery requires you to be an equal partner in the effort to treat your joints, not just the passive recipient of your doctor's care. Start keeping a record of the various treatment options your doctor discusses, and what each will mean for you and your life. You will want to discuss these options with your family and employer later, and it's important for you to be prepared for these important discussions.

EDUCATE YOURSELF

Aside from talking with your doctor, educate yourself when you start to think you may need surgery. Learn everything you can about making the decision to have surgery and what is involved in the process. Read about different surgical options for arthritis – reading this book is a great start.

Make sure that you understand all of the potential risks and benefits of joint surgery. Any type of surgery, including joint surgery, is serious business and should not be undertaken lightly. As with any surgery, there are risks involved. We'll go over these risks in more detail later in this book. But before you decide to have surgery, you should know that this procedure and the recovery afterward require a physical, mental and emotional commitment from you. You'll need to prepare yourself in all of these aspects. And you'll need to make sure that you can commit yourself fully to doing whatever it takes to make your operation and recovery successful. Use this book as a guide to help you do just that.

You should also talk to other people who have had joint surgery, especially people whose symptoms and affected joints are similar to your own. Ask about how they made the decision to have surgery and what the experience was like for them. You may find out about some aspect you hadn't considered before that makes surgery more or less appealing as a treatment option for you. Being as educated as possible about the prospect of surgery and everything that is involved will help you feel more comfortable in making your choice.

Common Joint Surgeries

Each year, more than 260,000 knee replacements and about 160,000 hip replacement operations are performed in the United States. Arthroscopy is also a very common joint surgery: About 1.5 million arthroscopic knee surgeries are performed each year.

Dispelling the Myths About Surgery

When thinking about surgery, many people feel apprehensive not only in making the decision to have surgery, but also in the weeks leading up to the procedure. These feelings are, of course, normal. People may have many misconceptions about surgery and what their bodies will be like after the surgery. Let's try to clear up some of those misconceptions here.

Surgery is a serious consideration because there are risks involved, including the challenges of getting through the recovery period. Will you be able to get around your house, use the bathroom or take care of yourself after the surgery? Will you be able to put up with the daily recovery exercises you will need to perform in order to get well? Knowing what you are about to face is the most important component of pre-surgery preparation.

Many people are also fearful of **anesthesia** and the risks that procedure can bring. These risks do exist. But we will try to discuss the important questions you should ask your doctor about anesthesia so you will be more informed about it. Plus, many people express the uncertainty of not knowing how they'll feel after the operation or how long it will take before they feel like themselves again. They fear that the surgery may not do enough to reduce their pain and increase their mobility, and their quality of life will always be diminished.

Give yourself a break! These fears about surgery are all understandable.

There's good news: A great deal of fear and uncertainty about joint replacement or other types of joint surgery can be alleviated with information and education, and in open, honest discussions with your doctor about the operation. Other big parts of alleviating those fears is having a surgeon that you feel confident in and that you trust and in having everything in place for your recovery before your operation. This book will give you advice on finding a surgeon you feel comfortable with and on all the preparations you should make before your surgery date. Knowledge and preparation should alleviate most of your fears, as well as the fears of your family.

In addition, many fears may be based on myths and misunderstandings about joint surgery. Here are some of the common misconceptions about joint surgery and explanations of the reality. You will see that medical advances have made this procedure much more successful for many people with joint problems like arthritis.

Myth One:

I'm too young for joint surgery. Some people believe that they are too young to have joint surgery, particularly joint replacement surgery. In the past, some people with joint pain or other problems, like arthritis, may have been told this by their doctors. They believe that they will have to endure their pain for years until they have reached an age when such surgery is appropriate for them. Where does this idea come from?

In the past, typical joint replacement parts lasted for between 10 and 15 years. So years ago, many surgeons were reluctant to perform joint replacement surgery in relatively young people or in those who have not been severely affected by pain and decreased mobility. The reason is that younger people are likely to be more active and mobile after the operation, and they would far outlive the life span of the new joint. The surgery would then need to be performed again once the replacement joint wore out. Many surgeons were opposed to the idea of performing a surgery in a patient that would have to repeat the procedure a decade or so later.

Now, however, advances in medical technology have improved the durability of artificial joints so that they last longer. New materials for joint replacement parts and new techniques for adhering those parts to the joint itself have also improved the quality and stamina of these replacements. In addition, doctors are considering joint replacement sooner for younger patients who can enjoy the benefits of a more active lifestyle as a result of surgery. A number of high-profile, very active young people – such as former professional athlete Bo Jackson – have had successful joint replacements at a young age, helping to alleviate some of the fears about joint replacements and activity level.

Myth Two:

Surgery will cure my arthritis. Joint surgery is a therapy used to help relieve some of the symptoms of arthritis, but it is not a cure for arthritis. Unfortunately, there is no cure for arthritis at this time. There is more information about controlling arthritis in the resources section at the end of this book. While joint surgery can help ease pain and improve your ability to move and function, surgery will not affect the disease process of osteoarthritis or rheumatoid arthritis, or other common arthritis-related diseases.

Even if you do have joint replacement surgery or other types of joint surgery, you will still have to self-manage your arthritis through maintaining a healthy weight, staying strong and flexible through exercise, taking medications that your doctor may prescribe and keeping up with your overall health. Even after joint surgery, you probably will experience some degree of pain and limited mobility, and you may still need to take some medications when necessary.

The fact that surgery can't cure arthritis is a factor in the decision to have surgery for many people with progressive forms of arthritis, such as rheumatoid arthritis. Because the disease will continue to affect the body after surgery, it may influence the benefits someone with rheumatoid arthritis will experience from joint surgery.

Myth Three:

You go in for the operation and come out feeling good as new. Wouldn't that be nice? Actually, having any kind of surgery, especially joint surgery, is quite an involved endeavor and not an easy one at that. That is what this book is all about: Helping you to understand what's involved in having joint surgery and what you'll need to expect from yourself in order to make it work.

Joint surgery involves time, money and a commitment to making it work. You'll need to make preparations before surgery and carefully follow your treatment and recovery program afterward. Surgery can help reduce your pain and improve your range of motion in a joint. But remember: Even after the operation, your joint will still not be the same as it was before you developed arthritis or had your injury. But a successful surgery may greatly improve your mobility and well being, enabling you to be more active and able to engage in things you may have given up due to your pain. The greatest factor in achieving that goal is you. If you are willing to put in the effort to do your exercises, maintain your healthy weight and stick to your physical therapy routine, your chances of having a long-term improvement in your joint are much greater.

Myth Four:

I'm too old for joint surgery. Some people mistakenly believe that if they're older, they can't have joint surgery, particularly joint replacement surgery. They may also believe that they are at increased risk for complications just because of their age. They may think they that their age will prevent them from withstanding the anesthesia involved in surgery or the recovery efforts afterward. Or they may simply think that age alone prevents them from being a good candidate for the surgery.

But that isn't necessarily true. Your overall health and ability to withstand surgery and recovery are more important considerations than simply your age. In fact, healthy older people are not at any greater risk from surgery than younger people are. They also have an advantage in the fact that they are less likely to outlive the joint replacement, needing another operation when the replacement joint wears out.

The most important point to take from this discussion is that you should not assume you are either too old or too young for a joint operation – ask your doctor what he or she thinks and, if necessary, consult an orthopaedic surgeon on your own to get another opinion on your candidacy for joint surgery.

Myth Five:

If I decide to have joint surgery, I have to have a total joint replacement. Total joint replacement is an option for people with severe pain and mobility limitations from advanced arthritis, but it is by no means the only surgical option that can help.

Your orthopaedic surgeon can discuss a number of other surgical options with you, some of which may be more appropriate for your specific case. Some options are also less invasive than total joint replacement.

There are some new procedures in joint replacement that involve smaller incisions and require much shorter recovery time. Arthroscopy of the knee is often very helpful in relieving pain and improving mobility. Be sure to ask your doctor if there are other types of surgery you should think about other than total joint replacement.

The right time to have surgery is not clear cut and the same for everyone. The decision to have surgery is an individual one. Each person has his or her own tolerance for pain and mobility problems that can affect the ability to enjoy daily life. There is no clear answer to when the right time is to have surgery. That is a decision you need to make on your own with your doctor's help. It is based on the severity of your arthritis and how much it affects your daily activities. While it may sound like a cliché, you will probably know when the right time is for you. You're likely to feel ready when you have reached your limit for coping with the effects of severe arthritis and need further relief that other methods no longer provide.

QUESTIONS TO ASK YOURSELF WHEN CONSIDERING SURGERY

Before you decide to explore surgery, however, it is important to have a discussion with yourself and with your doctor. Because surgery has risks and requires a major commitment from you, joint surgery is not necessarily for everyone. You'll need to assess your need for surgery, your ability to withstand the demands involved, and your ability to handle surgery's emotional aspects. To help you in your discussion with yourself, we've provided some questions below that you can ask yourself as you contemplate exploring joint surgery.

- Can I bear the pain that I am experiencing now, or does this pain significantly limit what I'm able to do?

- Have I given up all or most of the activities I enjoy because of pain and other arthritis symptoms?
- How much does my pain limit my movement and my ability to get around?
- Has my pain and stiffness increased steadily over the past several months to a year?
- Am I prepared for working through the recovery process from surgery, including post-surgery exercises and physical therapy if necessary?
- How will surgery help my condition? What realistic level of improvement can I expect following joint surgery?
- Are drugs, exercise and other therapies failing to provide the adequate relief that they have in the past?
- Does my insurance policy fully cover joint surgery and recovery costs, such as at-home nursing care if I need it? Are there out-of-pocket costs that I will have to bear? Can I afford these costs?
- Will I be able to take the necessary time off to recover from surgery? Will my family and/or loved ones be able to help me if I need them during my recovery?

LOOKING AHEAD

In this chapter, we have introduced you to the concept of joint surgery. We've looked at some of the reasons that may lead you to consider joint surgery, as well as some of the personal considerations you'll need to explore before you decide to have surgery. The rest of this book will examine in more detail the process of surgery and recovery, as well as the mental and physical preparations required for surgery. Next, we'll look more in depth into why you may need to have surgery and how to begin discussing the option with your doctor.

chapter 2:

Why Would You Need To Have Joint Surgery?

As you begin to think about the possibility of surgery, you're probably hoping for any treatment that will help you feel better. You're struggling with joint pain and with the difficulties you face in performing everyday tasks. You're probably frustrated that you've been unable to find anything that helps.

At the same time, surgery may still seem to be a frightening prospect. No one wants to have surgery unless absolutely necessary. Some people are afraid of the procedure itself, of undergoing an incision and of feeling pain afterward. You may be wondering if you can really withstand the operation and recovery. And you may be apprehensive because you still don't know what to expect from surgery, or even how to go about considering it. Simply put, surgery is daunting.

In this chapter, we'll help you through these concerns by helping you to understand the consideration of surgery a little better. We'll look at some of the reasons behind why you would need to have joint surgery. You will gain a better understanding of the conditions behind a need to have joint surgery and how these can affect your life. You will also understand what happens to joints in order to make surgery necessary.

Reasons for Having Joint Surgery

Joint surgery is often done to help correct joint problems that make moving difficult or painful. We discussed this a little in the first chapter. These joint problems can result from a number of different causes, such as a hereditary defect, injury or an illness that affects the joint. Any of these problems can cause pain or difficulty moving that may require joint surgery to correct the problem. While these conditions may make joint surgery necessary, one of the most common reasons for surgery is a condition called arthritis.

The word arthritis literally means "joint inflammation." (*Arth* means joint; *itis* means inflammation.) Arthritis is a very common disease – more than 43 million Americans have some form. But arthritis isn't a single disease – it is an umbrella term to mean any of the more than 100 diseases and conditions affecting the joints. As we learned in the last chapter, osteoarthritis (or OA) is the most common form of arthritis. It is also known as "degenerative joint disease," because it involves the gradual loss of **cartilage** (the smooth, rubbery substance that covers the ends of bones in the joint and allows for proper movement) in the joint. There are many other forms of arthritis, including rheumatoid arthritis, ankylosing spondylitis and more. Some of these conditions are rare, but others are common and lead many Americans to seek surgery as a treatment.

WHAT IS A JOINT?

Arthritis affects your joints, the places where two bones meet. The joint has a structure of its own, and several parts. There are several different types of joints. The type of joint, its location and the type of damage that has occurred in the joint all factor into any surgical treatment you and your doctor explore.

Joints are found all over your body: Your knees, hips, fingers, toes, ankles, wrists, shoulders and elbows all have joints. In fact, there are nearly 150 joints all over your body, linking your 206 bones. There are more than 70 movable joints in the body. They allow our bodies to be flexible and make almost any type of movement possible.

There are several different types of joints. They differ in their construction and in how they move. Let's go over a few of the types of joints in your body now:

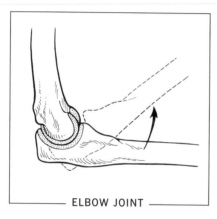

ELBOW JOINT

Hinge joints, such as knees or elbows, move back and forth like the opening and closing of a door's hinge.

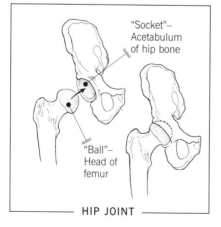

"Socket"–
Acetabulum
of hip bone

"Ball"–
Head of
femur

HIP JOINT

Ball-and-socket joints, like the hips or shoulders, consist of a bone with a ball-shaped ending that fits into a round socket. This construction lets the bones twist and turn in many directions while staying in place. However, as you may be aware, they can be dislocated in falls or accidents.

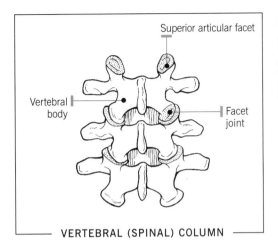

Superior articular facet

Vertebral body

Facet joint

VERTEBRAL (SPINAL) COLUMN

Facet joints, like those in the spine, allow the bones to twist, turn or rotate for a broad range of motion.

Basically, a joint is where two or more bones meet. Covering the ends of those bones is cartilage, a strong, smooth, elastic tissue. Cartilage acts as a shock absorber for your joints, and allows the joint to move smoothly. When cartilage becomes thin as in osteoarthritis, the bones at the ends of the joints can rub together, causing pain whenever the joint is moved.

The entire joint is enclosed in a **joint capsule** composed of tough connective tissue and lined with a thin membrane called the **synovium**. The synovium secretes a viscous, or slippery, liquid called **synovial fluid**. This fluid lubricates the joints, making movement easier.

Supporting your joints are **muscles**, soft, fibrous tissues that surround and support your joints and help move the joint. Also surrounding the joint are **tendons**, which are thick, cordlike fibers at the ends of muscles that connect them to the bones; and **ligaments**, which are supporting tissues that attach to bones and help keep them together at a joint. Fluid-filled sacs, called **bursae,** are next to tendons and ligaments and help cushion the supporting structures of joints.

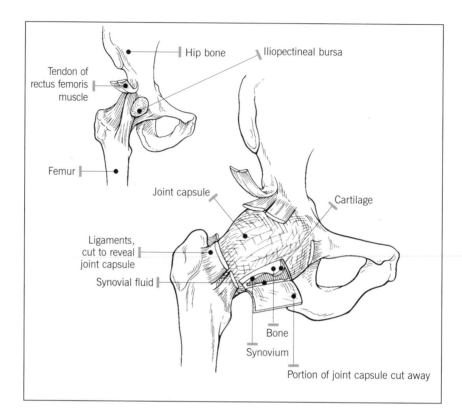

Depending on the particular injury, disease or problem you have, almost any of these structures – from the bone, cartilage and synovium inside the joint to the ligaments and tendons that support the joint – can be affected.

Because of their structure and the fact that they have moving parts that rub against each other all the time, many joints are subject to arthritis, especially osteoarthritis, the "wear and tear" type of arthritis. Of all the forms of arthritis, osteoarthritis is the most common reason for having joint replacement surgery, although many people with rheumatoid arthritis and other forms of arthritis and related diseases also have these surgeries, even in multiple joints.

COMMON TYPES OF ARTHRITIS

Many people who are considering joint replacement surgery don't realize that the pain they are experiencing is due to this very common disease. "I don't have arthritis; I just have to get my knees replaced because they are worn out and I'm in pain. But I *don't have arthritis*," they may say. You may be saying the same thing!

The fact is they probably do have osteoarthritis. They may say they have joint pain, joint stiffness, trouble moving their joints, bad knees/hips/elbows or some other description. But their doctor probably will tell them, if they ask, that their symptoms are due to osteoarthritis. While osteoarthritis is a chronic condition with no real cure, the good news is that there are many treatments, including surgery, that are effective at relieving their pain. Let's learn more about osteoarthritis and other forms of arthritis now.

Osteoarthritis

Osteoarthritis is the most common form of arthritis, affecting approximately 21 million Americans. The disease typically sets in after age 40 and it most often affects women. Osteoarthritis results from years of wear and tear on the joints that cause the breakdown of cartilage, the shock-absorbing, elastic material in the joints. Cartilage covers the ends of the bones and absorbs the shock of day-to-day movement. When cartilage begins to wear away and break down, the ends of the bones are left to rub together, resulting in pain and stiffness in the joints. This pain can often be excruciating. In many people, it simply can't be eased by aspirin or other common medications.

As we noted, osteoarthritis is a common reason that people have joint surgery, particularly joint replacement surgery. In addition to surgical procedures to replace the entire joint component, other surgical procedures may be used to treat problems associated with osteoarthritis.

In some cases of OA, pieces of bone and cartilage can break off due to the deterioration of the joint. These pieces can float loosely inside the joint, causing pain. Arthroscopic surgery may be required to remove these loose pieces of material and help relieve pain. If OA severely damages a joint so that little cartilage is left and the bones rub against each other, total joint replacement surgery may be needed to replace the damaged joint with an implant that will function similarly to the original without the pain from OA damage.

Rheumatoid Arthritis

Another common type of arthritis is **rheumatoid arthritis**, which affects about 2 million Americans. Rheumatoid arthritis (also known as RA) may affect people in their 20s and 30s, as well as older people, and it tends to affect more women than men. This type of arthritis is known as an **autoimmune** disease.

What is an autoimmune disease? The body's immune system is designed to fight off foreign invaders, such as infections and diseases. But in an autoimmune disease, the immune system mistakes the body's own tissues for foreign invaders and attacks them. In rheumatoid arthritis, this means that the immune system attacks the joint tissues, causing inflammation, swelling, pain and stiffness.

Over time, inflammation can damage the joints, causing weakness and even deformity in some cases. Inflammation eventually can cause the joint to change shape so that the structures that make up the joint are out of place for proper functioning. Fingers, for example, may drift to one side of the hand so that it becomes difficult to grasp items or even to straighten the fingers.

Joints severely damaged and misshapen by RA may require total joint replacement to allow comfortable, proper movement again. In fact, this type of surgery is common for people with RA and often helps them regain movement in these joints. Other types of surgery, such as **synovectomy**, can be used to remove diseased joint lining to help relieve pain.

Ankylosing Spondylitis

Ankylosing spondylitis (AS) is a type of arthritis that usually affects the spine or back. Joints and ligaments that normally allow the back to move in various directions become inflamed. Pain and stiffness result, usually starting in the spine, neck and hips, impairing mobility.

Over time, the disease can progress upward, causing problems in the upper back, chest and neck. As a result, joints and the bones of the spine, the **vertebrae**, can become rigid and unable to move. Other joints, such as the shoulders, can also become inflamed in AS.

Joint replacement surgery can be an effective treatment for some joints affected by AS, such as the hips and shoulders. Complex spine surgery can sometimes be used to treat the spine problems associated with AS, but this procedure is not widely performed. For more information on back surgery, consult *All You Need To Know About Back Pain: Beat Pain, Increase Your Mobility, Know Your Options,* published by the Arthritis Foundation. This book is available for $19.95 by calling 800/207-8633, or on www.arthritis.org. The Arthritis Foundation also has free information on ankylosing spondylitis, including a pamphlet you can request to have mailed to you, on its Web site.

HOW ARTHRITIS HARMS JOINTS

Arthritis is usually a progressive disease, which means that it continues to get worse, especially if you don't receive treatment. Many treatments, such as medications, are designed to slow down the progression of arthritis. Even with treatment, in many cases the disease can gradually advance. Joints may deteriorate to the point where you cannot perform ordinary tasks and live your life normally.

Depending on the type of arthritis you have, the disease can harm your joints in some slightly different ways. As we learned earlier, osteoarthritis causes the cartilage in your joint to break down and wear away. Cartilage is important for providing shock absorption and cushioning in your joints as you move. This breakdown destroys part of the structure of the joint that allows it to function properly. The actual shape of the joint changes as cartilage wears away.

The breakdown of cartilage also makes it difficult for the joint to work as it should. Joints are sophisticated structures that are designed to work precisely. Swelling, inflammation and cartilage damage can push the joint structures, such as bones, out of place. A swollen knee becomes stiff or a torn piece of cartilage doesn't cushion against impact as it should, making it difficult for the joint to move through its range of motion smoothly. Surgery may be necessary to drain excess fluid from swelling or to trim away a jagged piece of cartilage that is causing pain. In some cases, a procedure such as total joint replacement may be necessary to completely replace a joint in which cartilage and bone are damaged severely.

Inside the joint, osteoarthritis causes other changes, as we learned. Loose fragments of bone and cartilage can float in the joint fluid and cause irritation and pain. Bony **spurs** may develop on the ends of the bones, and the joint fluid may not be able to absorb shock properly. In some cases inflammation can occur in the joint lining as a result of the cartilage breakdown. Surgery can be used to replace a damaged joint in which the cartilage and bone are affected greatly. An artificial joint will have the proper cushioning to allow smoother, pain-free movement.

In rheumatoid arthritis, an autoimmune disease, the process is slightly different. Remember that this form of arthritis causes swelling and inflammation in the joint, which can lead to joint damage. The lining inside the joint may become swollen and inflamed from the body's immune response. The inflammation can damage the cartilage in the joint and erode the bone itself. Bone rubbing on bone due to the lack of cushioning cartilage, as well as inflammation can lead to terrible pain and lack of mobility.

Joint surgery can be used to ease pain by replacing damaged portions of the joint, so that there is once again proper cushioning for impact. A joint that was practically impossible to use can become mobile once again.

OTHER REASONS FOR JOINT SURGERY

While arthritis is a common reason that many people have joint surgery, there are other reasons that someone may consider joint surgery.

People may injure their joints in an accident, fall or sports activity. Many athletes (not just professional sports stars, but ordinary people engaging in sports or outdoor activities) can damage their joints due to an injury or simply through repetitive use.

In addition, consistent use of joints through very ordinary activities may lead to problems later on that require surgical treatment. Certain work tasks or sports may require repeated movements over and over for long periods of time. Here are some examples of these activities. You don't have to avoid them entirely, but ask your doctor if these activities could be contributing to your pain.

Sports That May Lead to Joint Injuries

- Tennis
- Golf
- Football
- Basketball
- Baseball or softball
- Running or jogging
- Skiing
- Soccer
- Gymnastics
- Ballet or other forms of dance

Work Activities That May Lead to Joint Injury

- Stocking shelves
- Typing
- Manual lifting
- Packing or unpacking boxes
- All-day standing or walking (in retail or warehouse setting)
- Landscaping
- Operating heavy equipment
- Construction
- Data entry

These are just a few of the many activities that may lead to joint injury if there is repetitive strain on certain joints. Without the proper equipment, body position or rest periods, these repeated movements eventually may cause what are known as **repetitive strain injuries**, damage to joints, and even osteoarthritis.

In addition, trauma, such as from a major injury or an event like a car accident, can seriously damage a joint. This type of impact may result in permanent damage. The joint may be misaligned from the trauma so that it no longer moves the way it was designed to. Over time, moving in an improper way can wear away cartilage faster than usual. This type of injury can lead to a condition like osteoarthritis years later. You may not even remember a particular event that led to your joint problems.

What caused the damage doesn't really matter once the damage exists – treating the problem is the most important thing. However, you may be able to help prevent OA or joint injuries from occurring by modifying your activities – for example, by wearing the appropriate footwear when you run or stretching out properly before you exercise, or by using the right techniques to do heavy lifting or other manual labor. Your doctor or physical therapist may be able to advise you on ways to reduce the risk of injury or strain to your joints. If you have arthritis, consult the book *Tips for Good Living With Arthritis,* available by calling 800/207-8633 or online at www.arthritis.org.

Many people, whether a person doing routine activities or a highly active person participating in sports, face injuries to their joints on a regular basis and may require surgery. In some people, that surgery may be needed right away to repair the joint and help heal the damage properly. In other cases, the joint may be injured by the individual may not seek treatment right away. After months or years, though, an injury such as torn cartilage can continue to cause pain. To relieve the pain, surgery may be needed to remove the damaged portion of cartilage and to determine if there is any other injury to the joint.

Some other reasons for joint surgery include diseased bone or **bone tumors**. A tumor is an area of tissue that forms when cells divide in an uncontrollable manner. It can be benign (non-cancerous) or malignant (cancerous). Tumors can appear anywhere in the body, including in or on bones and joints. A surgeon may perform surgery to remove the tumor and surrounding tissue from the bone or joint, and in some cases, replace the removed bone or joint with a transplant or artificial replacement (prosthesis).

So many situations can lead to a need for joint surgery. Surgery can help ease the pain of arthritis or repetitive strain injuries by repairing the joint. Damaged pieces of cartilage or loose pieces of cartilage or bone that can cause pain inside a joint can be removed or trimmed through surgery to provide relief. Surgery can also help to reposition a joint knocked out of place by the trauma of an accident or injury. This repositioning can allow the joint to function properly and relieve pain from misalignment.

Whether you seek surgery due to arthritis, a joint injury or other condition, it's important that you have a thorough discussion about your prospects with your doctor. Let's look at how you can create a successful pre-surgery dialogue with your doctor now.

How To Discuss Joint Surgery With Your Doctor

In the last chapter, we told you how to open the discussion of your joint pain and other problems with your doctor. Surgery is one of many options to consider for treating your problems. Your doctor will be a valuable partner in your search for pain relief and, if you choose to have it, in your journey through joint surgery. You'll need to communicate well together so that you can find the best and most appropriate option to meet your needs. And because surgery is a lengthy and challenging process, you'll need to trust your doctor and feel that you can rely on him to give you the best care.

The type of doctor who typically performs joint surgery is an **orthopaedic surgeon** (see below). An orthopaedic surgeon will work together with your health-care team to supervise your ongoing treatment and care. This team consists of several professionals who will work with you – you are an important part of your own care – to help you through preparation, surgery and recovery.

Your Health-Care Team

Think of all the doctors, nurses and other health-care professionals you see as a baseball team – everyone has a role to play. If everyone works together in sync, you'll be a successful team! You have an important position to play too. You're the general manager and coach of your health-care team – you pick the players and manage all the relationships and interactions between the various team members. If you stay involved in the process, you will improve your chances of success.

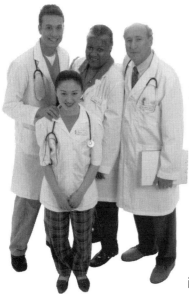

Who's on your health-care team? Depending on your situation, the roster may vary a bit. But here are some of the types of health-care professionals that will probably be recruited to play on your team.

Primary-Care Physician

A **primary-care physician** is your regular doctor. This professional might also be called a general practitioner, family physician or an internist. This is the doctor you see for a wide variety of ailments (including the flu or a backache). This doctor may diagnose the problem (such as osteoarthritis) that leads to your surgery. Your primary-care physician can refer you to specialists, doctors who have extra training in specific areas of health care or who perform special functions in your care, such as surgery. You will want to keep your primary-care physician involved in your preparation and recovery from surgery, so he or she can be informed about your condition.

Orthopaedist or Orthopaedic Surgeon

An orthopaedist is a specialist with extra years of medical training in the treatment of bone injuries, problems and diseases and their treatment. An orthopaedic surgeon has specialized training in performing surgery on joints and bones. This is the doctor who will perform your surgery.

Rheumatologist

Rheumatologists have specialized medical training in the treatment of arthritis and related diseases. (The field of study of arthritis and related diseases is called **rheumatology**. These diseases are known as **rheumatic diseases**.) If you have arthritis, your primary-care physician may refer you to a rheumatologist at some point in your care. A rheumatologist might help identify and treat your arthritis and help determine if surgery is the best course of treatment for you.

Physiatrists

Physiatrists are doctors that specialize in physical medicine and rehabilitation. Physiatrists work with patients to restore function in the body through therapy, exercise, medical treatments and other methods.

Anesthesiologists

An **anesthesiologist** is a doctor who specializes in administering anesthesia during surgery. Anesthesia means drugs or chemicals designed either to numb portions of your body (known as **local anesthesia**) or cause you to go into a temporary unconscious state (known as **general anesthesia**) so you don't feel the surgical procedure. If you have surgery, your surgeon will work with an anesthesiologist that you probably will also consult with. This doctor plays a vital role in the surgery, for administering anesthesia (particularly general anesthesia) involves many risks, which we will discuss later on in this book.

Podiatrists and Podiatric Surgeons

Podiatrists and **podiatric surgeons** are physicians specializing in the treatment of feet, including arthritis that affects the foot. Podiatrists can prescribe medications, special foot supports and shoes. Podiatrists may also perform surgery to correct foot problems.

Nurses and Nurse Practitioners

Nurses are health-care professionals who assist your doctor in your treatment before, during and after your surgery. You will probably spend a lot of time talking to or being treated by a nurse during your medical visits, as well as during any hospital stay. Nurses can administer many tests, help you prepare for and recover from your procedure, and answer many questions for you. **Nurse practitioners** have additional training and are present in many medical practices. Nurse practitioners may examine you and make an early diagnosis. They can prescribe medications in some states. Some nurses may care for you in your home; such professionals may be hired through agencies for a fee. You may require in-home nursing care following your surgery, depending on your situation.

Physical Therapists

Physical therapists will be a key player on your health-care team if you have joint surgery. Physical therapists (or PTs) guide your rehabilitation and recovery process, helping you regain your range of motion, strength and flexibility. They can also suggest ways for you to build your cardiovascular health and control your weight, important factors in preparing for and recovering from surgery.

Physician Assistants

Physician assistants act as an assistant to a supervising doctor. The physician assistant might take your medical history, perform a physical examination, make a diagnosis and help you with ongoing management of your problem. Like nurse practitioners, they can suggest treatments, and prescribe drugs in some states.

Occupational Therapists

Occupational therapists specialize in helping patients find ways to perform everyday tasks with less stress and strain on your delicate joints. They can fit you with splints or other devices that help you perform ordinary tasks with less pain and stress on your joints. An occupational therapist (also known as an OT) may be able to help you with basic functions of your job, including computer work, office tasks or lifting.

Other Members of the Team

You may encounter other health-care professionals at other points during your surgery and recovery, including **pharmacists** who dispense your drugs and even **psychologists** or **social workers** who might help you deal with some of the emotional or work-related aspects of your procedure. It's important for you to communicate well with all of the health professionals involved in your care. They, in turn, will work together to make your joint surgery a success.

Communication: The Key to Successful Treatment

Communication is key in good health care. The doctor who manages your care, whether you have arthritis, have had a joint injury or other health problem, should be aware of how your pain, immobility and other symptoms are progressing. This health-care professional, whether it is your primary-care physician, orthopaedist or rheumatologist, should be aware of what you are doing to treat your pain and how your pain affects your life. If you can't speak openly to your doctor – if you are reluctant to discuss sex or other personal topics that may be affected by your pain, for example – finding a successful treatment will be difficult. You should know that your doctor is there to help you get better. If you truly feel uncomfortable talking to your doctor, you may not be seeing the right doctor for you.

Your rheumatologist or other doctor may be the person who first suggests to you the option of joint surgery. From there, he'll likely explain the benefits of surgery and how it can help you function and feel better. He may also refer you to the appropriate specialist to perform your surgery or supervise your recovery.

How do you start this conversation? We've already provided some questions you might ask yourself or your doctor about joint surgery. These questions can get the ball rolling in your discussion. If you feel that surgery is an option you want to consider, you may begin by explaining to your doctor how your arthritis or other joint problem is affecting your life. Describe any activities that you enjoy but can no longer do, or tasks at your job and in daily life that you have difficulty performing. Explain how arthritis pain affects your movements and tasks. For example, you might find that you can no longer mow the lawn regularly due to the pain in your knees. Describe how severe it is if you can. Your doctor may ask you to "rank" your pain on a pain scale or perform other tests to gauge the severity of your pain.

You may also ask your doctor for a status report on your arthritis and on how it appears to be affecting the joint that you want to consider for surgery. Basic diagnostic tests, such as **X-rays** (radiographic images of the inside of your joints), that your doctor may perform will be able to reveal some of this information. If your joint problem has not progressed to a point where your doctor feels it is necessary to perform surgery, you may wish to wait.

Ask your doctor to explain whether that joint will continue to worsen or whether he believes it has stabilized. Discuss other possible options to help ease your pain and improve your function. And be sure to describe methods you've tried and the outcomes you experienced.

LOOKING AHEAD

In this chapter, we have discussed the many conditions that may lead you to need or consider joint surgery. As we noted, joint surgery is a serious step, and most people explore non-surgical treatments to ease their pain and stiffness before trying surgery. Your doctor probably will recommend that you do the same, and suggest or prescribe various drugs and other treatments for your problems.

In the next chapter, we will look at the most common non-surgical treatments for arthritis joint pain. You may have tried these treatments, or you may wish to ask your doctor more about them. While surgery may be the appropriate next step for you, it is also important to know all your options for pain relief.

chapter 3:

Other Treatments and Preparation for Surgery

Because surgery is a more complicated and invasive option than other types of treatments, you should not rush into surgery before considering other methods for reducing your pain and increasing your mobility. Most people try a number of pain relief methods before opting for surgery. Here, we will briefly discuss the common, non-surgical treatments for arthritis and other joint problems, some of which you may have tried yourself.

MEDICATIONS

Most people with arthritis take some type of medication to ease the symptoms of the disease, including inflammation, stiffness and pain. People with rheumatoid arthritis may use strong, prescription-only medications, including **glucocorticoids**, **disease-modifying antirheumatic drugs** (known as DMARDs) and **biologic response modifiers**. These drugs may treat the symptoms or stop the progression of joint damage in people with RA.

While your situation may require you to take those drugs, in this section we will discuss more widely used drugs used to treat OA, including over-the-counter drugs that do not require a doctor's prescription. Remember: If you do take over-the-counter drugs to treat your pain or inflammation, tell your doctor what drugs you take and how much you take. It's important for your doctor to be aware of *all* the medications you are using, even those you buy without a prescription.

Medications used to control arthritis usually focus on relieving pain, but some newer medicines are targeting other symptoms and even disease progression. Your doctor will work with you to find the drug or combination of drugs that works best for you.

Analgesics

Analgesics are drugs that relieve pain. These medicines do not, however, relieve inflammation that can sometimes occur in OA. If pain relief is your main concern, these drugs tend to have fewer side effects than drugs that relieve inflammation.

The most commonly used analgesic is **acetaminophen**, which the American College of Rheumatology recommends as the first line of treatment for the mild to moderate pain of osteoarthritis. Acetaminophen is available over the counter as generic and store brands or as the name brands *Tylenol*, *Anacin* aspirin-free, *Excedrin* caplets and *Panadol*. Acetaminophen can be taken in doses of 325 to 1,000 mg every four to six hours, but no more than 4,000 mg should be taken per day. This drug can cause problems if used with alcohol. Check with your doctor before using acetaminophen if you consume more than three alcoholic drinks per day.

Ask your doctor if taking acetaminophen may be helpful for you. You should also discuss the appropriate dosage you should take, and if you should stop taking this medication prior to your surgery.

If you have very severe pain, your doctor may prescribe a stronger analgesic. Examples of stronger, prescription-only analgesics include propoxyphene hydrochloride (*Darvon*, *PC-Cap* and *Wygesic*), acetaminophen with codeine, and tramadol (*Ultram*). Often, these drugs are used only for short periods of time because they may carry the risk of drug dependence. Discuss this option with your doctor. Do not take any prescription analgesic that was not prescribed for you personally. If another doctor prescribed these drugs for you for another health problem in the past, do not take these drugs for your pain without consulting the doctor treating your arthritis or other joint problem.

Topical Analgesics

Topical analgesic medications include creams or rubs that are applied directly to the painful area. These products may be purchased over the counter without a doctor's prescription, and they may be very helpful if you have only a few affected joints or if oral medications alone don't help alleviate your pain. The most common active ingredients in topical analgesics are **counterirritants**, **salicylates** and **capsaicin**. Caution: Never use topical products with heat treatments, because the combination of the ingredients in these creams and heat (such as from a heating pad) can cause serious skin burns.

Counterirritants contain substances such as oil of wintergreen, camphor and eucalyptus oil. They stimulate nerve endings, distracting the brain's attention from joint pain. Some product examples are *ArthriCare*, *Icy Hot* and *Therapeutic Mineral Ice*.

Salicylates contain the same ingredient, salicylic acid, found in aspirin. Salicylates work in a similar way to an ingredient that is found in many oral medications. They hamper the activity of **prostaglandins**, which are chemicals in the body involved in pain and inflammation. If you are allergic to aspirin, check with your doctor before using topical salicylate products. Some brand-name examples are *BenGay*, *Aspercreme*, *Flexall* and *Sportscreme*.

Capsaicin creams contain the natural ingredient found in cayenne peppers. Capsaicin helps relieve pain by depleting a neurotransmitter that sends pain messages to the brain. Capsaicin products usually take a few weeks to work and can cause stinging sensations at first. Creams containing capsaicin are recommended by the American College of Rheumatology for treating pain associated with knee osteoarthritis. In addition to not using capsaicin creams with heat treatments, don't use them on areas where there is broken skin, and take care not to let capsaicin projects come in contact with your eyes. Some examples of capsaicin products include *Zostrix*, *Zostrix HP* and *Capzasin-P*.

NSAIDs

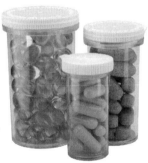

Nonsteroidal anti-inflammatory drugs, or **NSAIDs**, are a large group of medications used to help reduce joint pain, swelling and inflammation. You have likely taken NSAIDs at many times throughout your life, whether for a headache, a slight fever or sore joints.

There are several types of NSAIDs, and aspirin (*Anacin*, *Ascriptin*, *Bayer*, *Bufferin*, *Excedrin* tablets) is the most common. Other examples of over-the-counter NSAIDs include ibuprofen (*Advil*, *Motrin IB*, *Nuprin*), ketoprofen (*Actron*, *Orudis KT*, *Oruvail*), naproxen (*Naprosyn*, *Naprelan*) and naproxen sodium (*Anaprox*, *Aleve*). NSAIDs are available over the counter and by prescription. The dosage varies depending on the specific

Risk Factors for Ulcers or Stomach Problems

Stomach complications from NSAIDs can occur without warning, even in people who have never had stomach pain or heartburn. You may have a higher risk of stomach complications if one or more of the following risk factors is true. You may be at risk if you:

- Are over age 60
- Have severe disability from arthritis
- Smoke
- Have a history of ulcers or gastrointestinal bleeding
- Have a history of cardiovascular disease
- Consume more than three alcoholic drinks per day
- Use blood-thinning medications such as warfarin
- Use cortisone medications (prednisone)
- Are generally in poor health
- Have *Helicobacter pylori* (*H. pylori*) infection

drug. The drugs should be taken at the same time each day. If you have questions about which NSAID to take, or how often you should take them, ask your doctor or pharmacist. In most cases, generic or store brands of over-the-counter NSAIDs are the same as "name-brand" varieties that cost more. Ask your pharmacist about these products; you may save money by buying the store brand.

NSAIDs work by stopping the production of prostaglandins that occur naturally in the body, hormone-like substances involved in many body functions, including inflammation.

An important side effect to consider with NSAIDs, though, is stomach upset and irritation, which can eventually lead to stomach bleeding and ulcers. To guard against this possible problem, your doctor may recommend taking these drugs with food or taking a stomach-protecting drug as well. The stomach irritation associated with NSAIDs can be increased by alcohol consumption, so check with your doctor before using these drugs if you consume more than three alcoholic drinks per day. Also, if you are allergic to aspirin, check with your doctor before taking any NSAIDs.

COX-2 Inhibitors

COX-2 inhibitor drugs (short for cyclooxygenase-2 specific inhibitors) are a new type of more targeted NSAIDs. These new drugs include celecoxib (*Celebrex*), rofecoxib (*Vioxx*) and valdecoxib (*Bextra*).

Recent research has shown that there are two types of enzymes involved in prostaglandin production. One type, known as COX-1, produces prostaglandins that help protect the digestive system from its own corrosive acid. The other type, called COX-2, is involved in the production of prostaglandins that play a role in inflammation.

Traditional NSAIDs inhibit both COX-1 and COX-2, which not only decreases inflammation but also can cause damage to the stomach. COX-2 specific inhibitor drugs relieve pain and inflammation in a different way. Instead of affecting all prostaglandins, COX-2 drugs only stop production of prostaglandins involved in inflammation, without affecting those that protect the stomach (controlled by COX-1).

In theory, because they don't affect the stomach-protecting prostaglandins, the COX-2 drugs will be safer for the stomach than typical NSAIDs. They may be a good alternative for people who cannot take regular NSAIDs, or who have risk factors for serious upper gastrointestinal complications (see box on page 43). However, there is still the possibility of stomach side effects with these drugs, and they are considerably more expensive than regular NSAIDs. Check your insurance policy to make sure these drugs are covered.

Injectable Glucocorticoids

Glucocorticoids, also known as corticosteroids or steroids, are drugs related to the naturally occurring hormone in your body called **cortisone**. In some cases your doctor may inject these drugs into a painful joint for fast, targeted relief. For instance, when there is build-up of fluid in knee osteoarthritis, the doctor may drain fluid from the knee and then inject a glucocorticoid medication. You can only have glucocorticoid injections in the same joint three to four times per year because too many injections in a weight-bearing joint may possibly damage the cartilage.

Joint Fluid Therapy

A relatively new type of treatment specifically for knee osteoarthritis is known as **joint fluid therapy**. The treatment involves injection into the joint of **hyaluronic acid**, a substance found in the body that gives joint fluid its viscosity. This substance appears to break down in people with osteoarthritis. The injections are given once a week for three or five weeks, depending on the product (*Synvisc, Hyalgan, Supartz*). A small amount of joint fluid generally is removed first to make room for injecting the hyaluronic acid.

Clinical trials have shown that the injections may provide pain relief for people with mild to moderate OA of the knee. Relief can last for several months. It is not yet known whether the injections are helpful for other joints. So far, side effects include reactions at the injection site. Viscosupplement products just became available in 1998, so there is not yet a great deal of information available on the products' long-term effectiveness. Because of the makeup of these products, viscosupplement injections are not recommended for people who have allergies to bird feathers, bird proteins or eggs.

OTHER NON-DRUG THERAPIES

There are many treatments other than medications that you may try to ease your pain and other symptoms before considering surgery. Some of these treatments may be considered **alternative** or **complementary**, meaning that they are outside the realm of traditional medical treatments that your doctor would prescribe or supervise. No matter what treatment you try, make sure you tell your doctor what you are doing so he or she can assess your progress properly. Without all the facts, your doctor will not be able to see what is working and what is not working to ease your pain.

Here, we will briefly discuss some of the common non-drug treatments for joint problems such as OA. Again, ask your doctor if one of these options may be something you should explore.

Splints and Braces

Splints and braces, also called **orthotic devices**, can reduce pain and protect joints affected by osteoarthritis as you go about your daily activities. Splints can give your weak or unstable joints added support, or they can keep your joints in the correct position during certain activities and while you sleep. Splints and braces should be relatively affordable and easy to obtain.

While splints and braces may be helpful, your joints can become stiff if they stay in one position too long. That's why it is important to use a splint or brace only for a limited amount of time. You should also be sure that you continue to do appropriate stretching and other range-of-motion activities to keep your joints moving and prevent them from getting stiff.

An occupational therapist can design a splint or brace for just about any joint. Some splints are even available over the counter at medical supply stores, but you should still get a therapist's advice so you get one that fits properly and does what you need it to do.

Alternative and Complementary Therapies

Over the past several years, more and more people have become interested in alternative and complementary therapies. The reasons range from inadequate pain relief obtained from traditional therapies to an interest in natural treatments. Until recently, the term alternative medicine was used to describe all therapies outside of mainstream Western medicine. Now the more common term is complementary therapies, which refers to unconventional treatments used in conjunction with a traditional treatment plan.

Complementary therapies may:

- ease some symptoms, such as pain, stiffness, stress and depression;
- improve your outlook and attitude; and
- work with your medical therapies to enhance the effects of both.

You should neither expect complementary therapies to completely replace the rest of your treatment plan nor to cure your osteoarthritis or other joint problem. Instead, consider these therapies to be something additional you can do for yourself to take control of your condition.

Remember, even so-called "natural" therapies can have side effects or properties that could interact with the other medications you're taking. Discussing these therapies gives your doctor the opportunity to keep an eye out for any dangers or side effects you may experience. For more in-depth information on more than 90 alternative and complementary therapies for arthritis, consult *The Arthritis Foundation's Guide to Alternative Therapies,* available by calling 800/207-8633 or by logging onto www.arthritis.org.

Acupuncture. This centuries-old Chinese therapy is based on the idea that life energy called *qi* (pronounced "chee") flows through the body along clearly defined channels. According to this theory, illness results when qi is out of balance. Acupuncture uses very fine needles to stimulate points along those channels to put the qi back in balance.

How is acupuncture supposed to work? The scientific explanation for acupuncture's effect is that the inserted needles stimulate the body to release pain-killing chemicals called **endorphins**. Exactly how acupuncture works isn't yet clear, but it does appear to have very real effects in some cases.

Some studies indicate that acupuncture may be effective for osteoarthritis treatment. It may be useful for pain relief therapy in conjunction with medications. And if you are taking the medications only for pain, and not inflammation, acupuncture may allow you to reduce your dose. A consensus panel convened by the National Institutes of Health concluded that acupuncture can be an effective part of an overall osteoarthritis treatment plan. Ask your doctor if he thinks acupuncture is appropriate for your overall treatment. He may be able to recommend an acupuncturist for you.

It's important that you choose a qualified acupuncturist who is certified or licensed. Make sure the acupuncturist uses sterile, disposable needles.

Chiropractic. Chiropractic is an alternative treatment practice that involves manipulation and manual adjustment of the spine for the alleviation of pain and other symptoms. The practice is based on the idea that dysfunction in the spine can cause problems in other areas of the body.

Chiropractic may provide relief for some people. Manipulation of some joints may help relieve osteoarthritis pain, but you should be cautious because joint manipulation of weak or damaged joints could cause problems.

Chiropractic may not be safe for people who have osteoporosis or inflammatory conditions such as rheumatoid arthritis or ankylosing spondylitis. Be sure to tell any chiropractic practitioner about your condition and inform your medical doctor about your chiropractic treatment.

Vitamins. Researchers have found that certain vitamins, in particular those known as **antioxidants**, may help ease inflammation or pain associated with osteoarthritis. Antioxidants help destroy elements known as **free radicals**, which may contribute to OA. It is generally best to get vitamins from whole foods – such as fresh milk or oranges – rather than pills because the body seems to absorb and use the nutrients better this way. It is not advisable to take heavy doses of any vitamin as a way to "treat" your pain or other symptoms. This can be dangerous. Ask your doctor about the proper amount of any vitamin to take. A healthy diet of fresh, wholesome foods and the possible addition of a multivitamin supplement may be the best course for you.

Vitamin C appeared to counteract the wearing away of cartilage in studies of animals with osteoarthritis. In humans, this vitamin has been associated with decreased osteoarthritis progression and pain.

Vitamin E was shown to provide some pain relief in people with osteoarthritis in some studies. However, another study showed that it did not help ease osteoarthritis pain in African-American men.

Vitamin D may also play a beneficial role in osteoarthritis. One study found that progression of the disease was faster in people who had a low intake of the vitamin.

Herbs and Supplements

Looking at most health magazines and TV advertisements these days should prove to you that herbs and supplements are a booming business. Herbal remedies are increasingly available to consumers who want help for everything from depression to weight loss and even chronic illnesses like arthritis. And people are buying and using them in record numbers. A 1998 study by the Hartman Group revealed that sales of vitamins, minerals, herbs and other dietary supplements are around $10.4 billion a year.

Herbs and supplements are appealing to people with painful joint conditions like arthritis, for which there is no simple cure. In addition, some people with arthritis become frustrated by the seeming lack of relief that medicines such as NSAIDs provide in many cases. They are hopeful that so-called "natural" remedies will offer a gentler type of relief for their pain with fewer unwelcome and even dangerous side effects, such as ulcers.

Evaluating Alternative and Complementary Therapies

When you're considering a complementary therapy, be cautious. In your search for relief you may be willing to try something that holds little promise of helping your condition. In addition to the treatments that may help, there are also those that can hurt you or those promoted by people with little concern for your well-being who are only out for your money.

Be skeptical of therapies that:

- claim to work by a secret formula
- say they are a cure or a miraculous breakthrough
- are publicized in the backs of magazines, over the phone, or through direct mail – legitimate treatments should be reported in established medical journals
- rely only on testimonials as proof that they work

In addition, as you are considering an alternative or complementary therapy, keep the following advice in mind:

Most of these therapies are not regulated. Although drugs and other medical therapies are monitored and regulated by government agencies like the FDA, therapies such as herbs, supplements and some other alternatives do not have to undergo that type of scrutiny and are not approved by the FDA. So before you try an alternative treatment, learn as much as you can about it. A good source of information is the National Center for Complementary and Alternative

Medicine (NCCAM). For a free packet of information on alternative therapies, write to the NCCAM Clearinghouse, P.O. Box 8218, Silver Spring, MD 20807-8218.

Discuss the therapy you are considering (or already trying) with your doctor. Your doctor should be informed about any therapy you're trying, whether it is an alternative remedy or an exercise program. He can help you watch for and safeguard against side effects and possible negative interactions with medications you are taking. Your doctor can also answer important questions, such as how the therapy fits into your treatment plan and what precautions you should take.

If you proceed, do so with caution. Seek out a qualified practitioner. Practitioners of certain therapies are required to be licensed by a state or national board. If that isn't the case, find out about professional societies that provide certification.

Consider the cost and your coverage. Some alternative therapies can be costly. They may not be covered by your insurance. Examine your policy closely to find out what therapies may be covered and under what circumstances.

Use good judgment. If the practitioner makes unrealistic claims (such as, "It will cure your arthritis.") or suggests that you discontinue your conventional treatments, consider it a strong warning that something is not right.

Supplements offer the convenience of taking a pill or potion along with the idea that the organic ingredients pose little danger. But natural doesn't always mean safe. Some people think that supplements – especially herbs – are safer than the synthetic chemicals used in over-the-counter or prescription drugs. But herbs are chemicals too – anything with the potential to help your body could also be strong enough to hurt your body.

While most of these products may be unproven by formal medical testing or government sanction (herbal products are technically dietary products, and do not undergo the type of testing and scrutiny required of drugs) and even sometimes dangerous, others may provide some relief. Certain herbs and supplements have been shown to be helpful in treating some types of arthritis pain or inflammation.

Because of the increased use and interest in herbs and other supplements, researchers are beginning to investigate the effects and safety of these compounds to determine if the claims are valid – and if these products have a potential role in osteoarthritis treatment. For most herbs and supplements, there just isn't enough scientific evidence to draw a conclusion about their efficacy. There are few studies, and those that have been done don't stand up to scrutiny. As noted, the Food and Drug Administration does not approve these remedies, and they are not required to have the same safety and effectiveness testing that pharmaceutical drugs do. So it can be difficult to tell what you are getting.

Consult your doctor before deciding to try an herbal remedy or other supplement. And don't stop taking any prescribed treatments. Here's a rundown of popular supplements that may have some beneficial effects for osteoarthritis.

Glucosamine and chondroitin sulfate. Along with other complementary therapies, dietary supplements have gained popularity recently for treating a variety of conditions. Two that have received attention for arthritis treatment are glucosamine and chondroitin sulfate. These two substances are found naturally in the body. Glucosamine is an amino sugar that appears to play a role in the formation and repair of cartilage; chondroitin sulfate is part of a protein that gives cartilage elasticity.

A recent study of the two compounds funded by the National Institute of Arthritis and Musculoskeletal and Skin Diseases (NIAMS) and published in the *Journal of the American Medical Association* showed more evidence for the beneficial effects of glucosamine at the moment, but European studies showing the promise of chondroitin sulfate are mounting.

These two dietary supplements have been used for several years to treat osteoarthritis in dogs and horses, and in Europe to treat osteoarthritis in people. Studies done in Europe have found that people with mild to moderate osteoarthritis who took either supplement reported pain relief levels similar to those achieved with NSAIDs. They may produce a similar level of relief to NSAIDs, but take longer to begin working. Because few long-term studies have been done, there is little evidence of the supplements' effects over the long run.

The most common side effects of using glucosamine and chondroitin sulfate are increased intestinal gas and softened stools. Consult your doctor to discuss these other cautions:

- Women who are pregnant or who may become pregnant should not take glucosamine and chondroitin sulfate because the effects on unborn children have not been studied.

- If you have diabetes, get your blood sugar levels checked frequently because glucosamine may worsen your diabetes.
- If you also take blood-thinning medications or daily aspirin therapy, have your blood clotting time checked more frequently. Chondroitin sulfate is similar in structure to the blood thinner heparin and the combination has the potential to cause bleeding in some people.
- If you are allergic to shellfish, consult your doctor before deciding to take glucosamine because it is extracted from crab, lobster or shrimp shells. (But in most cases the allergies are triggered by the proteins in shellfish, and glucosamine is extracted from a carbohydrate called chitin.)

Most experts recommend trying supplements along with your regular medications for six to eight weeks. If you don't experience any change in your symptoms after a few months, then they are probably ineffective for you.

Avocado/soybean oil. Also called ASU, this is a mixture of these two oils that might ease osteoarthritis pain. Studies in France have shown some positive effects. This product isn't yet available in the United States.

Boron. This trace mineral helps the body use nutrients like calcium and magnesium. Boron eased osteoarthritis symptoms more than placebo in one study of humans. Some researchers believe boron has anti-inflammatory effects. Boron is found in many fruits, vegetables, nuts and dried beans.

What To Look For in Supplement Shopping

If you decide to try supplements like glucosamine and chondroitin sulfate, take care when choosing a product because supplements are not regulated by the FDA. Here are some other tips to help you:

- Choose products sold by large, well-established companies that can be held accountable for their products.
- Ask your doctor and pharmacist what they recommend. Take note of any side effects you experience and notify your doctor.
- Read the label to make sure the ingredient list makes sense to you. Ask the pharmacist for help if you have trouble.
- Choose products that say "standardized" on the label. Also look for "USP" on the label, which means the manufacturer has followed the U.S. Pharmacopeia's standards.

Boswellia. Boswellia is also known as frankincense. It comes from a tree in Asia. Some studies have found that when used with certain other herbs, boswellia may improve osteoarthritis symptoms.

Ginger. Ginger is a large, pale brown root found in many supermarkets. It is often taken in the form of tea or capsules as well. Ginger is purported to help relieve pain and inflammation.

SAM-e. Also called S-adenosylmethionine, SAM-e is a naturally occurring substance that may relieve pain as well as NSAIDs without the side effects. Some studies have also found it helps ease depression. Because folic acid plays a role in SAM-e production, you can increase your body's production of it by eating more green, leafy vegetables.

Hot and Cold Treatments

Hot and cold treatments are easy methods you can do on your own, at home or at the office, to reduce the pain and stiffness in your joints. Cold packs can numb the painful area and reduce inflammation and swelling. They are especially good for joint pain caused by a flare of arthritis. Heat, on the other hand, relaxes muscles and stimulates blood circulation.

There are many ways to apply heat and cold to your joints. You can try commercially available cold packs that can be placed in your freezer and refrozen as needed. You can make your own cold pack by wrapping a towel around a bag of frozen peas or corn, or a plastic bag filled with ice. Wrap the bag in a cloth or towel so the cold is not too extreme against your skin.

Heat may be dry or moist. Dry heat sources include commercially available heat lamps or heating pads. Ask your pharmacist to recommend a product that is right for you. Moist heat sources include warm baths, washcloths soaked in warm water or heated in a microwave oven (take care not to burn yourself!) and paraffin wax treatments, which involve placing the affected joint, usually those of the hand, foot, ankle or wrist, into a container of melted paraffin wax, which adheres to skin, giving warmth. These machines can be purchased at discount department stores or drugstores. Some brands include various types of scented wax and cushioned mitts. Shop around for the best price.

Tips for Using
Hot and Cold Treatments

Using heat and cold treatments can be an easy and effective way to reduce the pain, inflammation and stiffness in your joints. But there's a right way and a wrong way to use these treatments. To avoid burns or additional harm to skin and tissue, follow the suggestions below to get the greatest benefits from your hot and cold home treatments.

- Use heat or cold for only 15 to 20 minutes at a time.
- Avoid using treatments that are extremely hot or cold.
- Always put a towel between your skin and the hot or cold pack.
- Don't use creams, rubs or lotions on your skin with a c old or hot treatment.
- Turn off your heating pad before going to sleep, to prevent burns.
- Use an electric blanket or mattress pad. Turn it up before you get out of bed to help ease morning stiffness. Follow the directions on the blanket or pad carefully to ensure safety.
- Use a hot-water bottle to keep your feet, back or hands warm.
- Consult your doctor before using cold packs if you have poor circulation, or the conditions vasculitis and Raynaud's phenomenon.
- As with any treatment, follow the advice of your health-care professional when using heat or cold.

Before using either hot or cold, be sure your skin is dry and free from cuts and sores. If you have visible external skin damage, don't use cold or heat, especially paraffin baths. After using heat or cold, carefully dry the skin and check for purplish-red skin or hives, which may indicate the treatment was too strong. Allow your skin to return to normal temperature and color before using heat or cold again.

Water therapy. Everyone with sore or stiff joints or achy muscles probably knows how good it feels to soak in a warm bath, spa or hot tub (sometimes known as a *Jacuzzi*). It turns out that being in water not only feels good, it has real benefits for your joints. Studies have shown that the benefits of applying heat can include muscle relaxation and decreased pain and stiffness. Immersing your body in warm water is an especially good way to apply heat to many parts of the body all at once if you have back pain or pain in numerous joints.

If you find that pain and stiffness are worst in the morning, soaking and performing gentle exercises in a tub, whirlpool bath or warm shower upon arising can help you get ready to take on your daily activities. If pain increases throughout the day, a warm soak before bedtime might make it easier to wind down and go to sleep.

There are some exercises that may be performed in a hot tub or heated pool. To learn more, contact your local chapter of the Arthritis Foundation to learn about the Arthritis Foundation Aquatics Program, a series of exercise classes specifically designed for people with arthritis, led by trained staff and held in local swimming pools, including YMCAs (where the program is known as the Arthritis Foundation YMCA Aquatics Program, or AFYAP). You may also request a copy of the free brochure *Water Exercise: Pools, Spas and Arthritis.* Call 800/283-7800 or log on to www.arthritis.org to find your local chapter's contact information or to get this publication.

Massage therapy. Aside from medication, surgery and physical therapy, massage may be one of the most widely used treatments for sore, stiff joints associated with arthritis. Although the medical benefits of massage therapy for arthritis has not been extensively studied, many people report significant benefits in terms of reduced pain and increased relaxation.

Many doctors recommend massage therapy for their patients. Some doctors even have massage therapists working in their clinics, and your doctor will probably be able to recommend a massage therapist in your area. Although there are many forms of massage, the type most people are familiar with is **Swedish massage**, a full-body treatment that involves stroking or kneading the top layers of muscles with oils or lotions.

Other forms of massage include:

- **Deep tissue massage**, in which the massage therapist uses fingers, thumbs and elbows to put strong pressure on deep muscle or tissue layers to relieve chronic tension.
- **Neuromuscular massage** (also called **trigger point therapy**), in which the therapist applies pressure with the fingers to certain spots that can trigger pain in other parts of the body.
- **Myofascial release**, a type of massage that involves applying slow, steady pressure to relieve tension in the fascia, or thin tissue around the muscles.

Although massage therapy generally is safe, as with any therapy, there are some precautions. For example, you should never have mas-

How To Do Self-Massage

You walk through the garage and bump your elbow, causing pain. What is your first reaction? If you're like most people, you probably rub the painful area. And when you do, it probably feels a little better, at least for a while.

With practice, a similar type of do-it-yourself rubbing – called self-massage – can help relieve some arthritis pain. If you'd like try self-message, here are a few suggestions for getting started:

- **Get professional advice**. A licensed massage therapist can show you some techniques to use.
- **Warm up before you start**. A warm bath or shower can relax you, make your hands more limber and improve circulation.
- **Create a healing environment**. Find a warm, quiet place. Reduce distractions. For some people, soothing music can help create a relaxing environment.
- **Use a little lotion**. Using lotion can help your hands move easily over your body. A lightly scented massage oil can be soothing to your body also.
- **Consider an appliance**. If your hands are affected to the point where self-massage is painful or impossible, or if limited range of motion makes it difficult to reach painful joints, try an electric massage appliance. Be sure to follow package instructions and limit the use to a few minutes at a time.
- **Be firm, but gentle**. Use firm, gentle strokes and pressure, especially over the joints where skin and muscle layers are thin. Pressing too hard can irritate your skin and the joint or muscle you are trying to help.

sage on an inflamed joint or on skin that is broken or infected. Let your massage therapist know if you have other health problems, including circulatory problems.

If you think you might be interested in massage, consult your physician, physical therapist or other health professional who may be able to refer you to a massage therapist with experience in your particular condition. This massage therapist should be licensed by the local or state authorities governing massage therapy. Beware of "massage spas" advertised in small boxes in the sports section of your local newspaper or in the classified ads. These institutions may not be run by licensed massage therapists. Ask your doctor or physical therapist to recommend a reputable professional – your physical therapist may be licensed to perform massage also.

The Next Step: Choosing To Have Surgery

There are many new things to do when you have chronic joint pain and stiffness. And for your treatment plan to be effective, you have to follow it carefully and work with your health-care team. Write down the overall treatment plan you've discussed with your doctor and make sure you understand what you need to do and how it should help you. Be sure to discuss any questions you have or changes in your symptoms with your doctor.

If you've tried several of these methods or used some of them for a long time, your joint pain or stiffness may still worsen. You may find that you have to take larger doses of medication to achieve relief for your pain. This may concern you or cause unpleasant side effects, such as stomach upset. Or you may find that you can't get complete relief from medications or the other non-drug therapies we discussed in this chapter, and that the pain only gets worse over time.

As we noted earlier, you will know when you have had enough of pain and limits on your daily life. When you get to that point, you will know it's time to ask your doctor about the option of surgery. Ask your doctor if joint surgery is the best next step for you to take, and indicate that you'd like to know more about it.

CHOOSING YOUR SURGEON

Once you decide to explore surgery seriously, your primary-care doctor will refer you to an orthopaedic surgeon, as we discussed earlier in this chapter. You will have to find a surgeon who accepts your insurance plan. So bring your insurance listing of accepted or member physicians to your primary-care doctor visit or write down the names he or she recommends and look them up in the directory when you get home. Many insurance plans also have Web sites that list the surgeons they accept.

When you have a few names of surgeons recommended by your doctor and covered by your insurance policy, you may wish to ask people you know who have had joint surgery if they have heard of these surgeons. Recommendations from people you know and respect can help you choose the right surgeon. You may also wish to consider where the surgeon's office is located, what hospital they use for performing surgery, and what their office environment is like. We'll talk more about choosing the right surgeon for you later in this book on page 109.

Remember, surgery is a big decision! In the sidebar, "Ask Your Doctor About Surgery" on page 46, you will see a list of basic questions to ask your doctor prior to your decision to have surgery.

HOW TO TALK WITH YOUR FAMILY

When you are considering joint surgery, you should talk often with your family about what lies ahead. Your arthritis probably has affected the lives of other family members. Perhaps there are activities they enjoy doing with you (or tasks they need you to do) that you no longer feel able to do. They need to know that surgery may be a viable option for you. Discuss with them how joint surgery could help you feel better and perhaps make life better for the rest of your family as well. But they'll need to understand that during surgery and recovery, you will need a great deal of help from them just to perform basic self-care tasks.

Talk to them about how surgery will limit your activity for a while. Discuss the extra help and care you'll need from them during your recovery, and the amount of time that will take. And talk about the emotional support you'll need as well. Surgery can be a scary undertaking for many people. You'll need your family members to help you through this time as well as through the challenges of regaining your strength and mobility.

Find out what questions your family members have about the operation and consider taking one or more with you to a doctor's appointment so they can ask about any of their concerns. Be sure to share the literature and other information you have on joint surgery so they can better understand what will take place.

And because your recovery will take time and you'll need assistance, check with your family about the timing. If family members won't be available to help you or if another major family event is taking place soon, you may want to plan to have your surgery according to the availability of family members if possible.

Ask Your Doctor About the Surgery

The decision to have surgery is a big deal! So collect as much information as possible about the surgery before you agree to go through with it. But what do you need to know? Here are some important questions you may ask your doctor and/or the surgeon before surgery, so you will better understand the operation you are about to have.

You may also want to talk to someone who has had the type of surgery you are considering. If you don't know anyone, you may ask your doctor to refer you to one of his other patients who has had a similar operation. You can ask that person some of these questions, too.

Remember: Every person is different. Your problems may not be exactly the same as someone else's, even though the diagnosis is similar. Also, every surgery is different. Your surgery may not be the same as another person's operation. But it doesn't hurt to talk to someone who has gone through this type of procedure already.

Here are some great questions to ask your doctor or someone who has gone through surgery before to find out more:

- What other kinds of treatment could I have instead of surgery? How successful might those treatments be?
- Can you explain this surgical procedure, step by step?
- May I view materials or videos of this surgery?
- How long does this surgery typically take?
- Do you offer a class or informational meeting on the surgery?
- May I have this surgery on an outpatient basis?
- What are the risks involved in the surgery?

- Am I eligible for new, minimally-invasive techniques or high-flex replacements?
- How can I avoid blood transfusions? What other options are there?
- What type of anesthesia will be used? What are the risks of anesthesia?
- How much improvement can I expect from the surgery?
- Will more surgery be necessary? After what period of time?
- If I choose to undergo this surgery, will my family doctor be involved in my hospital stay? If so, in what way?
- Are you "board-certified"? Do you have a special interest or experience in arthritis surgery?
- What is your experience doing this type of surgery?
- Can you give me the name of someone else who has undergone this surgery and who would talk to me about it?
- Is an exercise program recommended before and after the operation?
- Must I stop taking – or increase the dosage of – any of my medications before surgery?
- What happens if I delay surgery? Even for a few months?
- What are the risks if I don't have the surgery?

Once you have asked some or all of these questions and you decide to have the surgery, you may wish to ask about the actual operation. What will happen when you are on the operating table? You will be curious to know this information.

Ask Your Doctor About the Surgery (cont.)

Here are some questions to ask your doctor or someone who has gone through this type of surgery before:

- How long will I need to stay in the hospital after the operation?
- How much pain will I experience?
- Will I get medication for the pain?
- What kind of pain is normal to expect? How long will this pain last?
- How long do I have to stay in bed while I am in the hospital? Or once I am home?
- When will I start physical therapy? Will I need to see a therapist in my home, or will I have outpatient therapy?
- May I see brochures or videotapes about recovery or rehabilitation?
- Will I need to arrange for some help at home? If so, for how long?
- Will I need to hire professional help, or will my family or friends be able to help me?
- Will I need any special equipment for my home? If so, what kind of equipment?
- Will I need to make any modifications to my home? If so, what kind of modifications?
- What drugs will I need during my recovery? How long will I need to take them?
- What activities should I not do during my recovery — driving, using the toilet, climbing stairs, bending, eating, having sex?

- How often will I have follow-up visits with you? Are these visits included in the cost of the surgery?

Some of your questions may have to do with your insurance coverage for this procedure. It's better for you to ask your insurance agent or company representative these questions rather than your doctor. Your insurance company can explain exactly what is covered and what is not under your coverage. If you are employed and covered by your employer's insurance carrier, there may be a person in your human relations department who specializes in your insurance coverage and can direct you to the right person at the insurance company to answer specific questions about what is covered. Ask your insurance company the following types of questions:

- Is this exact procedure covered by my policy?
- Am I responsible for any out-of-pocket costs or a deductible?
- What steps must I take before scheduling surgery?
- Is the hospital that my surgeon uses covered under my policy?
- Will any rehabilitation that I do in the hospital be covered by my insurance?
- Will rehabilitation that I do after I leave the hospital be covered by my insurance?
- Are the drugs I am likely to be prescribed covered under my insurance?

HOW TO TALK WITH YOUR EMPLOYER

Your decision to have joint surgery will also affect your job, including time away from work during your surgery and recovery. It's important that you discuss this matter with your employer well in advance of your surgery. You need to know your company's policies and what you need to do to make arrangements for your absence.

You'll need to check on your insurance coverage and find out about arranging time away from your job. Some employers may be hesitant about the impending surgery at first, because they will need to find a way to get your work done while you're away. But you should be positive and open with your employer about your decision. Explain how your current state of health – chronic joint pain, immobility, fatigue or other problems – affects your work life and how surgery might improve your situation.

Tell your employer that having this surgery is important to you and your well-being. Let him or her know that you are willing to do what you can to make sure your work gets done while you're gone. Describe how surgery can improve your ability to do your job and be a good employee in the long run.

You may also want to come up with some initial plans of how you can ease the transition and distribute your work while you are out having surgery. Efforts like these will show your employer that you care about your job and will take the time to make sure things go smoothly. Think of ways you can make the situation as easy on your employer as possible. And provide information on how long you will need to be away from work for recovery.

LOOKING AHEAD

In this chapter, we've introduced you to some of the treatments you can try before joint surgery. We've also looked at how you can begin discussing the details of surgery with your doctor and the people who will be affected in some way by your choice – your family and your employer.

Next, we'll explain the various types of joint surgery and the conditions they are used to treat. If you're considering surgery, there is more than one option available. We'll also learn which joints can be helped by surgery.

chapter 4:

What Are the Different Types of Joint Surgery?

While most people have probably heard of total joint replacement surgery, they may not realize that there are actually several different types of joint surgery. Total joint replacement is simply one of the most common procedures, and it may be the type of surgery that you will have. However, other kinds of joint surgery may be more appropriate for certain cases or to help alleviate specific joint problems.

Your doctor will be able to explain the procedure that is right for you, and discuss many of the specific details of the surgery you will have. To help you understand all of the options in joint surgery, this chapter will take a look at each type of surgery and the problems each is best suited to treat.

Types of Joint Surgery

There is one thing that all types of joint surgery, and all surgeries in general, share: They are serious procedures that carry risks as well as rewards. It's important that you know as much as you can before your operation.

We will touch on this issue later in the book. Now, let's examine some of the basic types of joint surgery and describe each procedure.

TOTAL JOINT REPLACEMENT (ARTHROPLASTY)
What is it?

In total joint replacement surgery, a damaged joint is replaced with artificial parts so that it functions more smoothly and with less pain. Replacement of hip joints was developed in the 1960s. Total joint replacement now is one of the most common and successful types of surgery.

What joints is it used for?

Many joints in the body can be replaced through arthroplasty, including hips, knees, ankles, toes, shoulders, elbows, wrists and fingers. The two most commonly replaced joints are the hip and knee.

Total joint replacement typically is performed when all conservative treatments, such as medications, exercise, and heat and cold, have failed to provide pain relief and improve function. Knee and hip replacements are common operations with high success rates as well, while replacements of smaller joints like fingers and toes can be a bit trickier. The precise movements and the small size of these joints make it difficult to create implants that work as well as the original joints or as implants for larger joint.

How is it done?

In arthroplasty, the surgeon makes an incision in the affected joint. He then cuts away at damaged or diseased bone or cartilage, resurfacing and reshaping the ends of the bones so the joint can be rebuilt. The surgeon then inserts a metal, ceramic or plastic artificial joint part, which is held in place either by a special cement adhesive or by the bone growing in around it. (See more on this procedure in the following pages of this chapter.)

Researchers and surgeons are making improvements all the time in artificial joint materials and surgery techniques. They are developing better materials that last longer, function better and have less risk of complications. Improvements in surgical techniques can improve the accuracy of implanting techniques, reduce the risk of complications, and perhaps even reduce the time it takes to complete the operation.

Types of Replacement Parts

The materials used in artificial joints vary, depending on the type of joint being replaced and how the joint needs to function. Hip joints, for example, need to be sturdy and able to bear your body's weight. Knee joints need to be flexible as well as strong, while finger joints must be capable of bending easily. In general, the components must be durable, flexible and able to function in the body without causing an immune system reaction.

Artificial joints have improved greatly since they were first introduced around 40 years ago. Replacements for hip and knee joints include portions made from metal, such as stainless steel, titanium, or chrome and cobalt alloys. Other portions are made of a strong, durable plastic called polyethylene.

There are new types of knee replacement parts that are highly flexible, allowing the knee to bend up to 155 degrees. Not all people qualify for such a component; ask your surgeon. The pieces are designed to fit perfectly together and to function as closely as possible to a natural joint. Special bone cement is used in some cases to hold static parts of the artificial joint in place.

Some new implants are made of a special type of ceramic material. These implants have an oxidized zirconium coating that keeps them from wearing out. While traditional implants last about 15 years, those made of the newer ceramic material can last approximately 20 to 25 years.

Traditionally, replacement parts for finger joints have been made from silicone, in order to allow the flexibility required of the fingers. However, this type of replacement has tended to slip somewhat because it does not fit tightly into the bones of the fingers. Researchers are working on new types of finger implants that are more like those used for knees and hips. These implants, like those for hips and knees, are made of metal and plastic materials that fit into the bones and more closely resemble a regular human joint. Researchers are still testing and perfecting finger replacements made of metal and plastic.

Cemented vs. Cementless Implants

In hip and knee joint replacement surgery, there are two types of replacements to consider: **cemented** and **cementless**, or a hybrid (combination) of cemented and cementless. The difference between the two types of replacements is in how they are held in place.

The cemented version, as the name implies, uses a special kind of bone cement that helps hold the components of the artificial joint in place. With cementless joints, the components that fit inside the bone are made of a porous material that allows the natural bone to grow into it.

Each type of implant has advantages and disadvantages. The cemented version may be better for older, less active people. That's because sometimes portions of the cement can break away, allowing the implant to loosen a bit. However, bone cement and surgical techniques have improved over the years so that cemented implants can work for younger and more active patients as well. Cementless versions may last longer in some cases, because there is no cement to loosen. However, these implants aren't a viable option for everyone. You need to have bones that are in good shape so they can grow into the prosthesis. (Cemented implants are generally a good choice for people with osteoporosis, a disease marked by porous, brittle bones.) Plus the recovery takes a bit longer than with cementless joints because the bone requires time to grow.

In addition, one version may work better than another depending on which joint is being replaced. Some surgeons also use a combination of the two methods of fixation. For example, some research has shown that cemented implants are more successful for knee replacements than the cemented version. In hip replacements, the cementless approach can work better for the acetabular portion (the upper part of your leg), while cement may be needed for the femoral component (the lower part of your leg). The combination is common in hip replacement surgery. In addition, there are new, minimally invasive knee procedures that may be used in some situations. They require less cutting and less recovery time.

How do you determine the kind of implant that is best for you? You'll need to talk with your doctor about the advantages and disadvantages of each one. Many factors, such as your age, weight, bone strength, the joint being replaced, and even the shape of your bones should be considered. Your doctor can help you decide which implant will work best for your body and lifestyle. Be honest with your doctor about your fears and concerns.

As we mentioned earlier, joint surgery doesn't just mean total joint replacement. There are many different kinds of surgical treatments used for joint problems. Some surgery is used for diagnosis, or exploring your joint to learn more about what is causing your pain or immobility.

In some cases one of these options may be better suited to treat your particular problem. When discussing joint surgery with your doctor, be sure to find out about all of your options. Also consult your insurance policy to see what procedures are covered. Let's go over these other types of surgery here.

ARTHRODESIS

What is it?

Arthrodesis is also known as bone fusion. The two bones that form a joint are fused together, and the joint is no longer able to move. This kind of joint surgery can help relieve pain and provide stability to the joint and help the joint bear weight more effectively.

What joints is it used for?

Arthrodesis typically is used for the ankles, wrists, neck, fingers or thumbs.

How is it done?

In this operation, damaged joint cartilage is removed, and in some cases, some of the nearby bone is removed too. Then screws or rods are inserted into the bones to hold them together. This holds the bones in place, allowing the joined bones to eventually grow together. The resulting joined bone lacks some of the mobility allowed by a moveable joint, but the procedure helps relieve pain and ensure stability of a damaged joint. This procedure can be particularly useful for ankles because joint replacement for this joint is rather new and its success is not yet established. Arthrodesis is the more common surgical option for this joint.

ARTHROSCOPY

What is it?

Arthroscopy (also known as arthroscopic surgery, a term you may be familiar with from your daily sports page, as many athletes undergo this surgery) is a very common surgical procedure in which a surgeon explores the inside of your joint by using an instrument called an **arthroscope**. The arthroscope functions like a tiny TV camera, letting your surgeon see the inside of your joint, magnified many times on a screen.

Surgeons use arthroscopy to make a diagnosis, to assess joint damage, to remove or repair damaged cartilage, and to smooth rough joint surfaces. Despite a recent study suggesting arthroscopy is ineffective in treating knee OA, it is useful for cleaning up loose particles, torn cartilage, or ligament and tendon damage in some patients' knees.

What joints is it used for?

Surgeons often use arthroscopy on shoulders and knees, but they are beginning to use it more for joints such as hips, wrists, elbows and ankles.

How is it done?

In arthroscopy, your doctor inserts an arthroscope and other tools through one or two small incisions in your skin. The arthroscope is a thin tube with a light at the end, and it is connected to a closed-circuit television in the operating room. The surgeon views the inside of the joint on the TV screen, identifying problems, such as loose pieces of cartilage or worn cartilage. Using other tools, the surgeon can then smooth out portions of rough cartilage or even remove floating pieces that are causing pain.

This surgery can be performed on an outpatient basis because it is less invasive than major surgery and requires a milder form of anesthesia. Patients recover from it more quickly than from other types of surgery, and they can usually walk with the help of crutches the next day. While arthroscopy can ease pain by smoothing the joint's surface or removing pieces of tissue that cause discomfort, it cannot change the progression of arthritis. Therefore, it may not be a permanent solution for some patients.

OSTEOTOMY

What is it?

Osteotomy corrects bone deformities through cutting the bone and resetting it in a better position. Misaligned joints can cause pain and can degenerate faster than normal joints because the bones aren't in the correct position to function properly.

What joints is it used for?

Osteotomy is usually performed on hips and knees to help relieve pain and allow the joint to function properly. Osteotomy may be used to improve the weight-bearing position of the lower leg in people with OA of the knee.

How is it done?

In osteotomy on the shinbone (tibia) or thighbone (femur), the surgeon reshapes the bone to improve the joint's alignment. In knee osteotomy, the surgeon repositions the joint to realign the leg so your knee glides freely and carries weight more evenly. He or she will then realign the healthy bone and cartilage in order to compensate for the damaged tissue in the joint. The surgeon will use one of several techniques to hold the joint in place while it heals, including a cast, staples or internal plate devices.

After surgery, the surgically treated bone can require several weeks to heal. Patients must also exercise and participate in physical therapy to keep the joint functioning during recovery.

Osteotomy may be a good choice for people who are younger than 60, active or overweight. Other criteria for good candidates include a lack of inflammation in the joint and uneven damage to the joint. The surgery can sometimes postpone the need for joint replacement surgery.

RESECTION

What is it?

Resection is a surgical procedure where a surgeon removes part or all of a bone. Resection is used to ease pain and improve movement when diseased joints in the feet make walking extremely difficult.

What joints is it used for?

Resection is used to remove **bunions** from toes, and also used on the wrists, thumbs and elbows.

How is it done?

In resection, the surgeon removes a portion of the bone from a stiff or immobile joint and creates a space between the bone and the joint. The bone does not grow back. Scar tissue grows in and fills the space where the bone was, offering more flexibility. However, the joint is less stable than it was when it was healthy.

SYNOVECTOMY

What is it?

Synovectomy is the removal of the diseased synovium, the joint lining that can become inflamed in rheumatoid arthritis, causing pain, swelling and disability. Removing the diseased tissue can help relieve severe pain and swelling and it can slow joint damage associated with rheumatoid arthritis.

What joints is it used for?

Synovectomy is used most commonly to treat the knees, shoulders, hands, wrists and ankles. Synovectomy is becoming less common in RA treatment due to the effectiveness of new drugs.

How is it done?

In synovectomy, the surgeon usually removes the diseased portions of the synovium using an arthroscope (see page 78), where he can see inside the joint through a tiny, tubelike camera that projects the interior of the joint onto a TV-like screen. For large joints, the surgeon may use a large incision in some cases. In time, the diseased synovium may grow back, leading to another synovectomy or possibly joint replacement surgery in the future.

LOOKING AHEAD

In this chapter, we've covered the many types of surgery that can be performed on a joint. We've looked at what is involved in these surgeries and what conditions they can treat. No matter what course you and your doctor decide to take, it's important to be aware of every option available to treat your pain or other symptoms. If you decide to have surgery, you and your doctor will discuss these options in detail and determine which one is most appropriate for your situation.

In the next chapter, we'll look at whether one of these surgical options may be right for you. We'll examine more closely what is involved in surgery and whether you may be ready to undertake it.

chapter 5:

Is Surgery the
Right Option for You?

Now that you have some more information on the types of surgery and what they involve, you may still be wondering if surgery is the right choice for you. Surgery is a serious consideration and it requires a long-term commitment to recovery. It is understandable that you may have hesitations and concerns.

Here, we'll try to address those concerns and help you think through the advantages and disadvantages of surgery, as well as the risks and benefits of forgoing surgery. While your doctor and surgeon can help you to better understand surgery and weigh your options, the ultimate decision is up to you.

Not Having Surgery – What's the Risk?

Although the decision to have surgery or not to have surgery is up to you, you'll want to take advantage of the medical expertise your doctor and surgeon have to offer. Your doctor has experience treating arthritis and he understands how it can progress. He can evaluate the status of your condition and the extent of damage to your joints.

In treating your arthritis, your doctor will likely first try medications, exercise and joint protection techniques to relieve your pain and help you move better. Once these methods stop providing adequate relief, however, your doctor may recommend surgery.

When your doctor recommends surgery, he is taking many factors into account. First, that your current treatment is no longer helping you enough. Your doctor is also aware of how your arthritis has progressed, and he knows what makes an appropriate candidate for surgery. In addition, he may have spoken to you about how pain and movement difficulties are affecting your life.

Part of your doctor's job is not only to treat your symptoms, but also to help you function as well as you possibly can. If you have reached the point where you need quite a bit of assistance from other people to manage simple daily tasks, and if you have stopped doing many of the activities you once enjoyed, then you and your doctor will see that you have had a major change in the quality of your life. Once arthritis has affected your life to this degree, you and your doctor may want to consider a treatment that can help you reclaim your former independence and activity.

One of the questions you should be sure to discuss with your doctor is what you can expect if you decide not to have surgery. Because surgery will require many major commitments from you, you should know whether having surgery is the right option for you. You probably already know that you can expect your pain and movement difficulties to continue. But will they stay the same, or will they become even worse? Are there more activities that you will probably have to stop because you can no longer do them? Will you require more and more help from friends and family to get through your day? Or is there a chance that your condition will stay as it is right now?

You'll also want to talk with your doctor about your candidacy for surgery. If you are an appropriate candidate for surgery now, is there a chance you won't be in the future? Will your arthritis cause damage that could prevent you from having surgery down the road? Do you have other medical conditions that could worsen and make it more difficult for you to recover from joint surgery if you don't have it now?

When you are considering something as serious as surgery, it is important to know if you could get by without undergoing the operation. Your doctor may tell you, however, that if you don't have surgery when he recommends it that your condition will continue to worsen. You may lose the ability to do other activities on your own.

By delaying, you may also run the risk that your arthritis may damage your joints to the point that surgery and recovery become more difficult. Your muscles can become weak from inactivity, so that the strength required for recovery becomes too much for you. If you have other medical conditions that grow worse, you also may no longer be a good candidate for surgery. Be sure to discuss all of these considerations with your doctor so you'll be aware of what you can expect to face without surgery.

REASONS FOR DELAYING SURGERY

When deciding whether to have surgery, both you and your doctor need to think about whether waiting to have surgery would be beneficial. Since you want everything to go smoothly during your operation,

Risks of Delaying Surgery

The following may occur if you delay joint surgery longer than recommended:

- Your condition may worsen.
- You may lose the ability to perform daily tasks on your own.
- Arthritis may worsen and damage your joints.
- Your muscles may weaken due to inactivity, making surgery and recovery more difficult.

there can be times when it is best to postpone surgery. Your doctor will be the one to decide if one of the following conditions makes it prudent to put off your joint surgery until a future date:

You may want to delay surgery if:

- You have an active infection, such as a cold, the flu, or a urinary tract infection, that needs to heal before surgery.
- You have another medical condition, such as heart disease or lung disease, that should be stabilized first.
- You don't have anyone who can help care for you during your recovery from surgery.
- You're overweight, and your doctor recommends losing weight before undergoing surgery.

Surgery Risk Factors To Consider

In addition to the reasons you may want to delay surgery, there are factors that can make surgery more risky for you. You'll need to think about these risks carefully. Talk with your doctor about ways you can moderate the risk and still continue toward your goal of pain-relieving joint surgery.

OTHER HEALTH PROBLEMS

If you have other health problems or chronic conditions, they can affect your ability to have surgery. Some conditions may need to be stabilized before you can be a good candidate for surgery, while others may present additional risks that your doctor and surgeon will need to take into account. Following are some conditions that can make joint surgery more complicated.

Osteoporosis

This disease makes your bones more porous and brittle so they aren't as strong as they should be. Depending on where osteoporosis affects you and which joint requires surgery, you and your doctor may need to make some adjustments. For example, osteoporosis can affect the type of implant your surgeon recommends. If your bones are very weak, a cementless implant may not be an option for you because the bone may not grow strong enough to hold the new joint in place. A cemented implant may work better for you.

Heart Disease

If you have heart disease or are at risk for it, your doctor may have you undergo a cardiac stress test before surgery. (Ask your primary-care doctor if you are at risk for heart disease. Risk factors for heart disease include smoking, excess weight, high cholesterol or a history of heart disease in your family.) A cardiac stress test will be administered by a cardiologist, or heart specialist.

A stress test indicates whether or not your heart can handle the stress of the operation. Surgery and anesthesia put additional stress on your cardiovascular system. Your doctor needs to make sure that your heart is strong enough to handle that added pressure and work. Also, blood thinners that you may take for a heart condition can make surgery more risky because they increase the risk of bleeding and prevent the blood from clotting.

If you have a heart condition, your doctor will carefully consider whether surgery is a good idea. Depending on your particular condition, you may still be able to have surgery. You may have to stop taking some medications in preparation for surgery or your doctor may have to give you alternate medications until after the operation.

Lung Disease

If you are a smoker or have a history of lung problems, your doctor will need to evaluate your lung function before surgery. The operation and anesthesia can be stressful to your lungs, so your doctor needs to be sure your lungs work well enough to overcome these challenges during surgery. Anesthesia puts additional pressure on your lungs, so weak or damaged lungs may not be able to withstand that additional stress.

Diabetes

If you have diabetes, your condition (including your glucose or blood sugar level, which often is elevated in diabetes) needs to be under con-

When It's Right To Say "Not Yet"

Here are the main reasons you may want to delay joint surgery:
- Active infection that needs to heal
- Serious medical condition that needs to be stabilized
- Lack of people to help you during recovery
- Excess weight that needs to be reduced

trol before you undergo surgery. Talk with your doctor about any special arrangements that need to be made to monitor your blood sugar during surgery.

Urinary Problems

Your doctor likely will test your urine during your pre-surgery medical evaluation, especially if you have had recent or frequent urinary infections. As explained above in the section about infections, urinary tract infections need to be treated before you have surgery. Any type of infection presents additional risks, especially in joint replacement surgery. You must be free of infections before you have surgery. Men who have prostate disease need to undergo treatment before having joint surgery. Talk to your doctor about your risk.

Excess Weight

Being overweight is bad for your joints, because it puts added pressure on the joints each time you move, eventually leading to damage over time. It can also make surgery more complicated. Sometimes, the surgeon has to make a longer incision (or cut) in the body of a heavier person. Added weight puts additional stress on your body on top of the stress caused by major surgery.

Excess weight can also make it more difficult for your surgeon to access the specific parts of your body during surgery and to be precise in his work. If you are overweight, it may be more difficult for you to do the rehabilitation exercises necessary to recover muscle strength after your surgery. If you are considerably overweight, your surgeon may recommend losing some weight before having joint surgery. Chapter 7 focuses on ways you might reduce your weight healthfully and maintain a proper weight for you. Maintaining your weight is an essential part of joint health, and will be important for you after your surgery and recovery.

Overall Fitness Level

Believe it or not, your fitness level can make a big difference in the success of your operation and recovery. If you are already in good shape before surgery, your operation likely will go more smoothly and you may recover more quickly because of your fitness level.

If you don't have an overall good level of fitness and if you have been inactive for a while, your operation may be more complicated. Surgery takes a heavy toll on your body, including your lungs, heart and muscles. If these organs are not in good condition, the stress of surgery may be too much for them. In addition, after surgery your mobility will be limited for quite a while and you will need to gradually regain muscle strength. If your muscles are already weak and out of condition, it may take you much longer to recover from a very limited activity level after surgery.

If your doctor determines that your fitness level isn't strong enough to make you a good candidate for surgery, he may recommend some ways to improve your fitness level and make surgery possible. This may mean you would have to put off surgery for several months while you work to improve your fitness level. Even if you are in enough pain to require surgery, there are still ways you can improve your heart and lung function. This may include activities such as water exercise, or if your legs are painful, vigorous upper body exercises done while sitting in a chair.

Medications –
What You Should Know

The medications you take for your arthritis and other conditions can affect your body during surgery. We discussed many of these medications in Chapter 2, but you may be taking other medications for other health problems, such as high blood pressure, high cholesterol, diabetes, heart disease or others.

In particular, medications that affect the blood's clotting ability can cause problems during surgery. These drugs include blood thinners, such as warfarin (*Coumadin*), and nonsteroidal anti-inflammatory drugs, such as the commonly used drugs aspirin (*Anacin, Bayer, Bufferin*), ibuprofen (*Advil, Motrin, Nuprin*), naproxen sodium (*Aleve*) and others. Talk to your doctor about your risk and even very common drugs you often take. If you continue using these drugs until the day of surgery, your blood will have less ability to clot and you may experience excessive bleeding during surgery.

To prevent serious complications such as this, your doctor will recommend that you stop taking these medications a few days to a few weeks before your operation. The timing depends on your dosage and how long the particular drug stays active in your bloodstream. Your doctor will give you specific instructions on when to stop taking your medication, and he can offer alternative pain-relief medications for you to use in the meantime. For example, acetaminophen (*Tylenol*) does not affect blood clotting and can be used up until the day of surgery. If you take blood thinners to treat a heart condition, your doctor may be able to recommend a different treatment.

There are some medications that you can continue to take until the day of surgery. Drugs such as methotrexate (*Rheumatrex, Trexall*) and prednisone (*Deltasone, Orasone*), often prescribed for people with rheumatoid arthritis, don't affect blood clotting and can be taken until the day of your operation. Ask your doctor if you should continue taking these drugs as you prepare for surgery.

KEEPING TRACK OF YOUR HEALTH CARE

If you see a number of doctors for different health problems, you will need to coordinate the information about your care very carefully. Your surgeon may need to be in touch with each of your doctors regarding your other conditions. And he will need to know all of the medications you take.

It's a great idea to compile all of your medical information in one place so that you can easily convey it to your surgeon. In a notebook, you may want to write down the names and contact numbers for all of your doctors, a list of the medications you take and for what condition you take them, and information about your insurance plan. That will make it easier to ensure that your surgeon has all of the information he needs about your overall health.

The Arthritis Foundation sells a ready-made health journal called *Health Organizer: A Personal Health-Care Record.* This spiral-bound, tabbed notebook has sections for keeping track of your doctors' names and contact information, insurance information, drugs you take, symptoms and actions you took to relieve them. To order, call 800/207-8633 or log on to www.arthritis.org to shop in the Arthritis Store. The Arthritis Foundation offers many products to help you increase your joint health and mobility, including books, brochures and videos.

Herbs, Supplements and Alternative Treatments

As we discussed in Chapter 3, alternative treatments – also known as complementary treatments or therapies – can include everything from herb and supplement pills to topical creams to acupuncture. More and more people with joint pain use these treatments, which do not require a doctor's prescription.

Herbs and supplements, which may be purchased at grocery stores, pharmacies, on the Internet or in natural health stores, are not tested or approved by the Food and Drug Administration (FDA), as drugs are. Therefore, their quality and effectiveness are not substantiated. However, herbs and supplements and other alternative treatments can have powerful effects on the body, so it's important to keep track of what you take.

You should always keep your doctor informed of any supplements or alternative treatments you're using, especially when you are preparing for surgery. Although these therapies are touted as "natural," they still contain strong, active ingredients. Sometimes, the ingredients listed on supplement labels are merely other names for more familiar ingredients, including stimulants and depressants.

These ingredients can potentially interact with other medications you take, and they can also affect your body in other ways. Like some of the drugs you may be taking, some supplements may affect the clotting ability of your blood. Supplements can have other effects that you may not be aware of, so be sure your doctor knows what you are taking so he can advise you when to stop taking it before your operation, if necessary.

INFECTIONS

Infections are an important concern in any type of surgery, before and after the procedure. They are a danger that can make the operation more complicated and the recovery take longer. In joint replacement surgery, infection around the implant can be very serious, and can even require that the implant be removed so that it can be replaced with a new one. Having one surgery requires enough time, energy and recovery; you don't want to have to have another surgical procedure soon after your first one.

As noted earlier, before surgery, your doctor must make sure that you are free of infections so that it does not compromise the success of your surgery or cause additional dangerous complications. Your doctor will evaluate you with tests to confirm that you have no infections, including urine tests to check for bladder infections. Your doctor may also recommend that you have a dental evaluation to check for oral infections. An infection anywhere in your body could make its way to the site of your surgery. If you do have an infection, your doctor will treat you with antibiotics to heal the infection before you have surgery. Be forthright with your doctor about any recent infections you have had and what course of treatment you used.

ARRANGING FOR RECUPERATION TIME

The type of joint surgery you have affects your recovery time. Therefore, the amount of time you have to be away from work or other normal activities depends on what procedure you are having. Less invasive procedures, such as arthroscopy, have relatively quick recovery times that can allow you to go back to work within a few days. Major surgery, though, such as total hip or knee replacement, takes considerably longer.

After some joint operations, you may not be able to drive for a while. Your time away from work will depend greatly on what type of work you do. You may need to be at home recovering for six weeks or even up to 12 weeks before you can return to work. If your job requires a lot of activity or even lifting heavy objects, you may need to start back to work with lighter tasks at first. If you have a desk job that requires a long, stressful commute, getting back to work soon after your surgery may be difficult for you. You may ask your employer about a short period of telecommuting (working from home using your home computer, fax machine and telephone) or reduced work hours.

When you're considering surgery, discuss your recuperation time with your doctor. Be specific about the types of activities your job requires and the recovery time your doctor estimates you'll need. Get as much information and as many details as you can from your doctor so you can determine how long you'll need to be away from work. Then check on your company's policies regarding medical leave and insurance coverage for recovery. You will then need to talk to your employer about your need for surgery and for time away from work to recover.

Make sure you know your company's policies ahead of time and consider talking with your human resources department early on to confirm any coverage details. Emphasize to your employer that the time you spend away from work recovering ultimately will be worthwhile to them as well. The pain relief and improved function you experience will make you a better worker after your operation.

After talking with your employer, you may want to consider requesting confirmation in writing of the time you will spend away from work and the specifics of the arrangement. Talk with your employer about working ahead on some projects and getting help from co-workers to cover your responsibilities while you're away. Making this type of effort can put you and your employer at ease and help them to feel good about your time away for recovery.

Leave a contact name (perhaps a family member or friend) and number with your place of employment so they can contact you if necessary while you are out of work. Make sure your important projects are taken care of before you leave, or reassigned to a colleague if possible.

ARRANGING FOR HELP AT HOME

The help you'll need at home after surgery also differs depending on your type of operation. Arthroscopy and other less invasive techniques allow you to recover more quickly, so you'll need help getting home from the hospital and you may need someone to drive you where you need to go for a short period of time. If you are having total joint replacement of a knee or hip, or other more invasive surgical procedures, it might be necessary to get a friend, family member or even a hired nursing professional to help you get around your house and do ordinary self-care tasks, such as preparing meals and cleaning.

With major surgery like total joint replacement, your longer recovery period may mean that you will not go directly home after your surgery. You might have to spend some time in a rehabilitation center or a facility for short-term rehabilitation. Or, if you do go home after being discharged from the hospital, you might need more help at home for several weeks. You might have difficulty getting around for a while – even moving around your house may be a struggle.

At first, you may need assistance going to the bathroom, bathing and dressing. You'll need help preparing meals. And you'll need someone to drive if you need to go somewhere. You won't be able to lift and carry groceries until your hip or knee heals more fully, which will be several weeks. And you'll need assistance with chores around the house, such as cleaning, washing dishes, taking out trash. For the first couple of weeks, it will be a challenge for you just to get around the house, and you'll need help with that for the first few days or so.

As you make your other arrangements for surgery, you may also need to make arrangements to have help at home. Talk openly with your doctor about how limited you will be for how long. Discuss what types of activities you'll need help with. Depending on what type of surgery you have and what joints are operated on, tasks you'll need help with may include:

- Getting in and out of bed
- Bathing and/or showering
- Grooming
- Getting dressed and undressed
- Preparing your meals
- Laundry and basic housecleaning
- Transportation, including getting in and out of the car

Find out when family members and friends are available to help you. This may be an important part of your decision on when to schedule your operation. In addition, talk to your doctor or nurse about whether you need to consider hiring in-home care assistance for part of your recovery period. If you live alone or if your family members aren't able to help (or would have trouble managing required tasks), in-home care may be an option you need to consider. If you're the main caregiver in your household, in-home care may be especially important.

If you need to hire in-home care for the first few weeks after surgery, you'll need to talk with your doctor to assess just what you will need. Find out whether you need skilled nursing assistance or a home health aid. Home health aids may be covered by Medicare or other types of insurance coverage.

Depending on your type of surgery and your condition, you may not need the skill level of a nurse because you most likely won't need someone to handle complex medical monitoring. You most likely will need a home health aide who can help you bathe, dress, use the toilet, and help with cooking, cleaning and laundry. The cost is greater for someone more skilled who can handle more complex medical tasks. The fees are typically lower if you don't need that level of skill. Some health insurance plans cover this type of care to varying degrees. Be sure to check your plan carefully to find out exactly what type of care is covered.

You can find out about hiring in-home help through home health agencies. Check with your doctor or surgeon, or with the hospital where you'll have surgery, for contacts with local agencies that offer this service. It's important to do some homework before choosing a service. Talk with friends or family members who have had surgery and used in-home help for a referral. Before hiring any agency or person, check their references. You will want to feel totally comfortable with any outside person coming into your home to help you during this time when you will feel out of sorts.

Once you're home from the hospital, you'll be able to move around and take care of some of your basic needs. You may still need help, however, with some tasks, including running errands, getting groceries and cooking, doing laundry and carrying anything heavy. You will probably need assistance with these tasks for the first few weeks after surgery, so make arrangements ahead of time to make sure that family, friends or home health aides can be there to help you. Try not to put yourself in a situation where you will be helpless and not have anyone to assist you. It might be a good idea to put a portable intercom system in your recuperating room so you can communicate to your family member or helper in another room if you need immediate aid.

The Costs of Surgery

In addition to preparing mentally and physically for surgery, it's important for you and your family to prepare financially for the cost of the operation. Carefully check into your health insurance policy to find out what portions of the procedure they cover. If you have an insurance agent or a human resources representative at your office, discuss your procedure and your coverage before you schedule the actual surgery. Discuss any restrictions that apply, such as where you can have the operation or which surgeons you can see.

Most private insurance companies and HMOs, as well as Medicare and Medicaid, cover the cost of joint surgery. Be sure to find out what portion of your hospital stay, rehabilitation and other related costs are covered. Don't wait until you are recovering from your procedure to find out if you have any out-of-pocket costs – prepare well beforehand so you can be sure you can cover the necessary costs.

Talk with the staff that handles the insurance paperwork for your surgeon's office, your health insurance company and the hospital where you plan to have surgery to make sure you understand all of the costs involved. Talk to them about which portions your insurance pays and which ones you will be paying. It's important that they know who is being billed for various services. Ask for confirmations in writing so you can have documentation on hand if you need it, and so you can refer back to it if any discrepancies come up.

Here are some costs you should be sure to ask about when determining the total cost of your surgery:

- Surgery itself
- Any extra professionals brought in to assist the doctor
- Hospital stay (also find out the length of stay covered)
- Physical therapy (in the hospital and outpatient)
- Home health services
- Medications (including which ones are covered by the prescription portion of your insurance policy and if they come in generic form)
- Additional medical supplies, such as crutches, canes or hospital beds for home use
- Follow-up care or visits

If your insurance does not cover all of the costs related to joint surgery and recover, or if you don't have insurance, talk with your doctor's office about arranging a payment plan. In some cases you may be able to work out an agreement that allows you to pay in installments over time. But be sure you have everything worked out in writing before your operation.

As you plan for your operation, sit down with your family and your financial advisor to go over the costs. A financial advisor can help you get a realistic picture of all of the costs involved. Your family should also be aware of these costs. In addition, be aware that complications and other unexpected situations could result in additional costs. Talk with your financial advisor and your family about how you can plan for these costs and how you can estimate what they could be.

How much does a typical joint surgery cost? This number can vary greatly considering what type of surgery you are having, your doctor and where you live. On average, a typical total joint replacement surgery costs between $25,000 and $30,000. So you can see the importance of making sure you have discussed the entire procedure and all possible costs with your insurer beforehand! Insurance may or may not cover the cost of durable medical equipment, such as walkers, crutches or raised commode seats that you may need during your initial recovery period. Make sure you review your insurance policy carefully and ask a lot of questions if you have them. You won't want to have to haggle with an insurance company about covering an expensive item or procedure afterward, when you are trying to concentrate on getting your joint back into action.

LOOKING AHEAD

In this chapter, we've taken a realistic view of surgery, from whether it is the right option for you to the costs of the operation and other expenses. We've looked at factors that will determine whether you are an appropriate candidate for joint surgery and the practical concerns of medications you may have to discontinue until after surgery. We've also reviewed the planning you'll need to do for financing the operation and for the assistance you may need while you are recovering.

In the next few chapters, we'll focus in more detail on what you will need to do to get ready for surgery. We'll look at everything from how you can find a surgeon to how you can prepare yourself physically and mentally for the prospect of surgery.

"Going to the Hospital"

From *Celebrate Life: New Attitudes for Living with Chronic Illness*, by Kathleen Lewis, RN
Published by the Arthritis Foundation, 1999.

As you probably already know, if you have a chronic illness, you may to need to go to the hospital from time to time. Whether it's because of acute exacerbations of the illness, for re-evaluations, diagnostic work or for corrective surgery, you're probably not going to look forward to it with great joy.

Hospitalizations may make those around you suddenly more aware of your illness, even if the problems have been there all along. You may get a lot of extra attention, and your forces may rally to bring in food, take charge of the house, and hover over your children, which may embarrass them to death. Teenagers, especially, may want to shrink into the woodwork. Let them know that you're aware this experience is trying for them too, and allow them time to be with their friends.

You may find that going into the hospital bolsters your credibility of being sick with family, friends, health-care professionals or insurance providers. It's difficult for most people to realize that you can be ill while remaining functional and even cheerful.

You and your family's emotional, physical, and financial resources may be drained as hospitalizations turn family routines, schedules and budgets into chaos. All may be strained to meet the increased demands. Creating a plan with everyone who'll be involved can be helpful. Writing all the pertinent information down and leaving it in a central place can be helpful for everyone.

I have an emergency plan on the bulletin board next to the phone in my kitchen. I've included insurance information; important phone numbers including the doctor, pharmacy and vet; my list of medications; how to water the plants; etc. I try to consider anything that will need to be done in my absence. If you decide to write up such a plan, try to imagine what people would need to know to keep your household running in your absence.

If visits or phone calls from friends and family just add to the strain, be honest. Tell your support community what you and your family do and don't need to help you through this time.

BEFORE YOU GO
Negotiating the Details
Before a couple of my many surgeries during and after my divorce, my teen-age sons, Jamie and Keith, and I went to see the family therapist to negotiate my needs. I let them know that this was A BIG DEAL for me and I needed their support and help! They set boundaries on what they could and couldn't do for me.

They let me know that putting the whole community on alert about my illness embarrassed them. As teenagers, they were acutely and uncomfortably aware of being made to feel different from everybody else. At their ages, they most wanted just to blend in with everybody else. They also felt that certain people in our support community treated them like children and invaded our family boundaries too much.

However, as a single parent, I had certain responsibilities: I wanted to be sure the boys would never be alone in the house; that they were always to let me know where they were; and that they were to keep their same curfews. I recruited trusted friends and neighbors to help.

We even negotiated food needs. The boys felt if we bought a loaf of bread and a jar of peanut butter that we'd do just fine! I didn't buy their plan. We bartered on who would be asked to bring in food and what to tell them to bring. Yucky vegetable casseroles were banned.

The boys let me know whom they were comfortable with coming to stay with them. They were at an age where they only needed someone to check in with and serve as a home base.

Over the years, I found several people who'd come and stay at the house in my absence. My goal, with the help of my counselor, was to provide a balance of freedom and structure appropriate to their age whether I was in the hospital or not.

Jamie and Keith couldn't bear to visit me in the hospital. That would be the ultimate admission that their dad had left us and they were filling his role. They would call and check in on me. When I got home I knew to expect not TLC, but LLC (loud loving care).

I was determined not to cast the boys into any adult roles or fill duties their dad or other absent family members needed to assume. I didn't want adult roles thrust on them as they had been on me growing up.

My counselor, the boys and I negotiated that I would maintain expectations realistic to their age and their activities would be as undisturbed as possible. Jamie and Keith did find their own ways to be attentive and caring that really touched me. I found my counselor and family of friends to fill any adult roles needed.

Putting too much responsibility on teenagers of parents with illness, especially compounded by divorce, can interrupt their launching into their own lives. They may need to totally run away, act out in order to leave the home, or they may stay home and be rescuers. My boys seem to have launched pretty well, given all they had to go through in growing up.

Your children may wish to visit you in the hospital. If you would find that comforting, perhaps one of your support people could take them, and try to make it as unscary as possible. Explaining what the medical equipment is for and letting them see where you are may be comforting.

Realistic expectations of what we could expect of each other made hospitalizations, which could have been devastating, a growing experience in how to negotiate with each other. With the help of the counselor, we assertively, clearly and directly set our boundaries and asked for what we needed with "I" messages. WOW! What a difference!

Hospitality

Hospital procedures can be more unbearable than the condition that sent you there. Here are a few tips on how to make it through a hospital stay.

1. The medical directive NPO (an abbreviation for the Latin *non per os*; nothing by mouth) is often given for 12 hours before a lab test or procedure. It presents special problems for patients with a dry mouth or Sjögren's syndrome (a common disorder marked by dry mouth and eyes). Here are a few tricks:

    • Rinse mouth out with mouthwash or brush teeth, being careful not to swallow.
    • Suck a slightly damp washrag, letting dry mucous membranes absorb the moisture.
    • Apply lip balm.
    • Drink plenty of fluids right up to the time for NPO to begin.
    • Ask for a vaporizer.
    • Ask if you can be allowed to chew gum.

2. In prolonged visits, hospital sheets may rub your elbows raw. Putting alcohol on your elbows at the beginning of a stay to dry them out will make them tougher, and the sheets won't rub as much.

"Going to the Hospital" (cont.)

3.   To ease nausea:
  • Eat small, frequent meals.
  • Breathe deeply, from your abdomen.
  • Suck on ice chips.
  • Drink carbonated beverages or hot tea.
  • Apply a cold compress to forehead.
  • Eat dry toast or crackers.
  • Make sure the room is cool.

4.   Bring extra pillows from home to help position painful joints. When lying on your side, a pillow between the knees can prevent hip rotation. Use a pillow to support your arm and shoulder.

5.   Change bed position frequently to help alleviate back discomfort, sore joints or difficulty breathing. If you're having trouble breathing position the hospital bed so your head is up over halfway, and the knees elevated (if appropriate, considering the type of surgery you are having).

6.   Cheese crackers, if permitted in your diet, help take away bad taste of medications.

7.   Use cotton balls or earplugs to shut out hospital or roommate's noises so you can sleep.

8.   Dry hospital heat can dry out your sinuses. A vaporizer provides moisture and white noise to drown out other sounds.

9.   When pain or discomfort is intense, you'll be able to bear it better if you practice visualizing beautiful scenery or pleasant memories.

10. Isometric exercises (tightening and relaxing muscle groups), wiggling toes, flexing muscles, and deep breathing exercises (even while confined to bed) can help promote relaxation and increase circulation. Ask your nurse or a visiting physical therapist if these type of moves are OK for you.

11. Some hospital procedures require lying still in uncomfortable positions for long periods of time. Try:
    - Focusing on points in room to provide a diversion
    - Wiggling toes or any part of the body in a rotating manner
    - Or anything that would help you focus away from lying still

12. Whether or not you have circulation problems that leave you with cold hands and feet, take extra blankets and several pairs of socks. Layers work best. Hospital temperatures can be cool. Emergency and operating rooms will actually heat blankets for you.

13. Remember to take your journal or books. Writing can pass time, as well as release anxiety about what you are going through.

In the age of managed care, hospitalizations are shorter and less frequent. Make the most of your stay. Once again, make it business, write down your observations and questions, and remember you're the one who is ultimately responsible for you.

*To order a copy of **Celebrate Life**, call 800/207-8633 or log on to www.arthritis.org.*

chapter 6:

Getting Ready for Surgery

Now that you've made the decision to move ahead with joint surgery, you'll get into the details of preparing for your operation. At this stage, there are many more choices you'll need to make about exactly how you want your operation to proceed. These choices include which surgeon will operate on you, what type of anesthesia you'll have, and where the surgery will take place.

In addition, you'll need to get to work preparing yourself physically and mentally, as well as at work and home, for your operation. In this chapter, we'll take you through all of these choices and the many preparations you'll make before your joint surgery. Being properly prepared for surgery is one of the most important things you can do to try to make your surgery and recovery as successful as possible. Mental preparation is a key component also, and we'll discuss how to get your mind ready for surgery, as well as your body, finances and family.

How To Choose Your Surgeon

One of your first decisions will need to be choosing your surgeon. Of course, your particular medical plan may determine some of your choices. Be sure you understand the details of your plan and how its coverage levels are affected by the surgeon you choose.

Some plans may pay more of the costs if you choose a surgeon on their list, while they may pay a smaller percentage to none at all if you choose a doctor not on the list. Find out if your insurance company requires special documentation from your primary-care doctor or specialist for you to be treated by a surgeon. If you are covered by an insurance policy provided by your employer, you may ask the human resources manager to explain this aspect of your policy to you.

REFERRALS AND RECOMMENDATIONS

In addition to checking with your insurance plan, you may want to get recommendations and referrals of surgeons to consider. Your primary-care doctor or rheumatologist, if you're seeing one, should be able to give you a list of recommendations. You should also ask people you know who have had joint surgery to recommend someone to perform your surgery. Friends and acquaintances are a good place to get honest referrals.

You will also feel better by being able to ask about the experience they had as patients. How a patient is treated by their surgeon encompasses more than just the surgery itself – it also includes how the surgeon answers questions, interacts with the patient and makes the patient feel involved in the process.

Another source of recommendations for surgeons is a physical therapist. Physical therapists often work with joint surgery patients after surgery, so they are familiar with surgeons who perform the operations, plus they get the patients' perspectives as well. Usually, when you are in the hospital the PT on staff will work with you to supervise your initial recovery. If you require a physical therapist to work with you once you are discharged, you may want to look for a PT who specializes in joint replacement rehabilitation. Consult your insurance policy to learn what physical therapy services are covered. You can ask your doctor for the names of physical therapists who work on post-surgical rehabilitation in your area.

PROFESSIONAL ORGANIZATIONS

Along with referrals from other doctors and from friends, you may also want to check into professional organizations that can give you some help. Some organizations have lists of physicians in your area while others can provide records of their certifications. Arthritis Foundation chapters have lists of local physicians licensed to perform joint surgery.

The American Academy of Orthopaedic Surgeons can give you a list of their members in your area. Explore their website at www.aaos.org. Membership in the organization means that the surgeon likely keeps up with the latest research and techniques in orthopaedic surgery and that he is board certified in orthopaedic surgery. These organizations can also provide you with information to help you understand joint surgery and perhaps some questions to ask your doctor about surgery.

YOUR LOCAL HOSPITAL

Your local hospital can likely provide you with a list of surgeons who perform joint surgery at their hospital. The staff at the hospital may also be able to refer you to physical therapists that practice at the hospital. They also may be able to offer you the names and phone numbers of home health agencies you can contact for in-home care after surgery. Call the main number of the hospital and ask the receptionist to connect you with someone on staff who may be able to give referrals of surgeons, physical therapists or other professionals you need.

THE INTERNET

You can search the Internet for organizations that can provide referrals. You may also be able to find surgery centers and hospitals with web sites that offer information on their services and staff. You can also find organizations such as the American Academy of Orthopaedic Surgeons (mentioned on page 108) or the Arthritis Foundation to find out what services and referrals they offer as well as how you can contact them.

Here are the Internet addresses for several organizations that offer free information on surgery, arthritis, joint health, the latest medical research in these areas and more:

The American Academy of Orthopaedic Surgeons: www.aaos.org

The Arthritis Foundation: www.arthritis.org

The American Physical Therapy Association: www.apta.org

The American College of Rheumatology: www.rheumatology.org

The National Institutes of Health: www.nih.gov

American Academy of Physical Medicine and Rehabilitation: www.aapmr.org

The Bone and Joint Decade: www.boneandjointdecade.org

Centers for Disease Control and Prevention: www.cdc.gov

WebMD: www.webmd.com

To conduct your own search for information on your joint surgery, use some of the popular search engines on the World Wide Web. A few of these are www.google.com, www.yahoo.com, www.lycos.com, www.excite.com and many more. Some medical practices and hospitals have their own interactive Web sites that you can explore to learn more about doctors and other medical staff, as well as the facilities and services offered.

Questions To Ask Potential Surgeons

Once you have a list of potential surgeons, you will want to interview a few in person. An interview will give you the chance to see whether this is the right surgeon to perform your joint replacement or other surgery.

When you meet with surgeons to determine who will perform your operation, you will no doubt have many questions, not only about the doctor's background, philosophy and credentials, but also about the procedure itself. Mostly, you will make your decision based on gut feeling – how comfortable you feel with the surgeon's experience and approach.

It's important to find a surgeon you feel comfortable with, but you should also seek someone who has a good deal of experience performing the specific type of joint surgery that you'll be undergoing. Here are some questions you may want to ask prospective surgeons:

- Is the surgeon board certified in orthopaedic surgery? Board certification means that the surgeon has received training and passed examinations in a particular field of medicine, such as orthopaedic surgery or specific surgeries.

- How many times has he performed the type of operation that you plan to have?
- What have the outcomes been? Ask to talk with patients who have received this procedure from this surgeon and find out what their experiences and outcomes were like.
- Will the surgeon allow you to contact former patients to ask about their experiences?
- What are the most common complications and how does the surgeon propose to handle them?
- How can you reach the surgeon if you have questions or in an emergency?
- Who will be your main contact at his office? Who can help you with insurance questions?
- What is the surgeon's assessment of your condition and the most appropriate treatment?

The surgeon or his or her staff may also be able to provide you with materials such as booklets, brochures and videos to help you in understand the surgical procedure and in preparing for it. Ask your doctor about these materials as well. Also, find out if the surgeon can recommend any Web sites that may be helpful (see page 109 for more on finding health information on the Internet) as you prepare for your surgery.

HOW YOU SHOULD FEEL ABOUT YOUR SURGICAL TEAM

When choosing your surgeon, you should certainly consider credentials and experience as well as the referrals you've received. But in addition you should also consider your own feelings about the doctor.

Do you trust him? Do you have confidence in him? Do you feel comfortable with him and the care he will provide you? Do you like and feel comfortable with his nurses, assistants and office staff?

You should feel that the surgeon you choose is honest with you and will give you the best possible care. You should have confidence in his abilities to perform the operation and handle any complications. Remember, this is major surgery. You should also feel that the surgeon is accessible if you need him and willing to spend the time necessary to answer your questions and make you feel at ease with the procedure. You should feel this way not only about your surgeon, but also about the other members of your health-care team: physical therapists, nurses, anesthesiologist, and even the hospital where you'll have the surgery.

WHICH ANESTHESIA IS BEST FOR YOU?

The next important decision you will be making is which type of anesthesia you will have during surgery. To some degree the choice may depend on what type of surgery you're having, but it also depends on your personal preference. There are pros and cons for each type of anesthesia, but your surgeon will be able to advise you on your choice well before the day of your surgery, have a conversation with your surgeon and anesthesiologist about your options and which one may work best for your particular situation.

Let's discuss the different kinds of anesthesia now:

Regional Anesthesia

There are three types of anesthesia to choose from for joint surgery: regional, general and a combination of the two. **Regional anesthesia** uses medications applied through a catheter in your back to numb only the region of the body that will be operated on, while the rest of you remains normal and you are conscious of what is happening. The most common type of regional anesthesia used for joint surgery is called an **epidural**. Spinal anesthesia sometimes is used as well.

Regional anesthesia is administered through a tube inserted into your back so that the anesthetic is injected into the outer lining of your spinal cord. Spinal anesthesia is injected into the lower part of the back. The advantages of regional anesthesia are that you don't feel any pain during the operation, but you are otherwise awake and alert. In addition, recovery can sometimes be quicker with regional anesthesia because it doesn't require time and care to work the anesthesia out of your lungs and other body systems.

The **catheter**, a thin, flexible tube that allows fluids to be transferred into or out of your body, used for regional anesthesia can also be used to administer pain-relief medications after surgery. However, in some cases the regional anesthesia may not be completely effective and general anesthesia may have to be used.

General Anesthesia

General anesthesia, on the other hand, provides medication that puts your brain and whole body to sleep so that you feel and recall little of what goes on during the operation.

General anesthesia allows you to be asleep and pain-free during the surgery. The medication can be administered intravenously through a tube inserted into a vein or inhaled through a mask applied to your nose and mouth. Some patients find it more comforting to be unaware of the operation and then awakened when it is over.

The third option is a combination of the two approaches mentioned above. Regional anesthesia numbs the area of the operation while the patient is given a lower dose of general anesthesia to help him or her to relax and be less aware of the activity going on during surgery.

HOSPITAL FORMS

When you are admitted to the hospital for surgery, there will be a number of forms for you to fill out. These may be done on the day of surgery, or the hospital may have you complete them in advance. Some forms relate to **informed consent**. This term means that you understand the procedure you are about to undergo and the risks involved. These forms can seem a bit disturbing because they mention death as a possibility. This is a standard form and it is how the hospital makes sure you understand what the potential risks are and give them permission to treat you.

If you have any questions about the forms, be sure to have them answered by the hospital staff or your doctor before you sign them. Ask questions if you don't understand something in the forms! Don't be shy when your health, payment or liability is concerned.

Other forms give the hospital permission to give you medications for pain control. Some forms will spell out what you would like the hospital and doctors to do in case of an emergency (including contact phone numbers) or surgery complications, including how far you'd like them to go in resuscitating you if that need should arise. Again, don't be alarmed, but discuss these items with your doctor and your family members so that everyone understands what you are signing.

The purpose of these forms is to inform you and gain your consent for treatment. They also help protect the hospital and its staff from liability. Most forms should be routine for any type of surgery, but if you have any questions or don't understand something, be sure to ask.

YOUR HOSPITAL STAY

The length of your hospital stay will depend on the type of surgery you have, how quickly your recovery progresses, whether you experience any complications and what your insurance company covers.

Arthroscopy, for example, requires just a short stay to allow you to recover from the operation and the anesthesia. Patients typically go home from the hospital the same day. For joint replacement, however, your hospital stay can last several days. In most cases, patients leave the hospital after about four or five days. For more insight on preparing well for a hospital stay, see "Going to the Hospital" on page 102.

Preparing for Surgery

Before you have surgery, you'll need to take several steps to prepare yourself physically and mentally. Surgery is stressful to your body and mind, and you'll need time to recover. The steps you take ahead of time to prepare yourself can help you greatly in your recovery so that you can feel better more quickly. The surgery preparation advice covered in the following pages may not seem critical now, but if you follow it you will see how helpful it is.

WEIGHT LOSS

If you are overweight, your doctor may recommend losing weight before surgery. As noted earlier, this can help make the operation easier for your surgeon because it will allow easier access to the precise parts of your body he needs to reach during surgery. Losing weight can also help reduce the risk of complications during surgery and make recovery easier.

It is also important that you eat a well-balanced diet. During times of stress, such as surgery, it is vital that you get the proper nutrients you need. If you don't already eat a healthful diet, start now. If you need advice or recommendations, talk to your doctor or other member of your health-care team. In general, eat plenty of fresh fruits and vegetables, whole grains and small amounts of lean meat. Ask your doctor if there are any particular vitamins and minerals that would be helpful to your body during surgery. If you feel your diet is deficient, ask your doctor if a daily multivitamin supplement (available at all drugstores and super-markets) would help. Vitamin C may enhance the healing process, so ask your doctor if he thinks you should take a supplement or add certain foods containing the vitamin to your diet before surgery.

EXERCISE

Being in good shape can play an important role in your recovery. Because your body will be under stress from surgery, and because you will have to limit activity after surgery, you should make sure you're in good shape before surgery. Exercising before surgery can help strengthen your endurance and muscles so they can help you recover mobility and strength more quickly after surgery. You may also need extra upper body strength after surgery to help you use crutches to get around. Strengthening your upper body now can make your adjustment after surgery easier.

In addition, you will need to exercise after surgery to help in your recovery. You may want to practice and become familiar with the exercises that your doctor recommends now. Exercise can also help you lose weight if your doctor recommends it before surgery.

STOPPING SMOKING

Smoking can increase the risk of complications during surgery. If you smoke, you should try to quit or reduce the amount you smoke before you have surgery. Smoking also can slow down your healing and recovery. Exercise, an important component of your preparation for surgery as well as your recovery, can be more taxing and difficult if you are a smoker. Smoking is a general health danger.

PREPARING YOUR FAMILY

In addition to preparing physically for surgery, you'll also need to prepare your family to spring into action during and just after your surgery. Following your operation, you'll need time to regain your mobility and recover. You won't be able to move around as easily at first and will likely need help with many simple activities. You'll also need support and encouragement during your recovery, to help you deal with initial pain and to motivate you in exercising and regaining strength. Your family will play a very important role in your recovery.

Specifically, you'll want to designate one family member to be the contact person for doctors and other hospital staff during and right after your surgery. You'll also need a family member or friend to bring you home from the hospital and be with you for the first few days. Before the operation, your family may be able to help you prepare your home for your return from the hospital. They can also help you prepare meals ahead of time so you have quick, simple items that are easy to eat when you first arrive home.

Before your operation, discuss all of these issues with your family. Remind them that you won't be yourself for several weeks after the operation and that you won't be able to do the things you usually do until you recover.

PREPARING YOURSELF

Perhaps your biggest job before surgery will be preparing yourself, both physically and mentally. Here are some of the things you may want and need to do before surgery that will help you feel in control of the process and ready for your operation.

Understand the procedure. Be sure you have thoroughly discussed the operation with your doctor and surgeon. Make sure that you understand exactly what will take place, as well as how you will feel afterward. (We'll go through the surgery step-by-step in Chapter 9.) If you have any questions, clear them up before your operation so you feel at ease with what will take place.

Take a class. To help patients feel more comfortable with joint replacement surgery, many hospitals and surgery centers offer classes to help patients prepare. These classes are taught by health-care professionals and patient educators who review all of the steps of surgery with you. They also offer helpful advice on preparing for surgery and on getting through the recovery period successfully. The instructors can answer your questions and help allay any lingering fears or uncertainties you may have. Find out if your medical center offers these classes and consider taking one before your surgery.

Review your medications with your doctor. Some medications can affect how your body reacts to surgery, including its ability to heal and the blood's ability to clot properly. As noted earlier, nonsteroidal anti-inflammatory drugs, including aspirin, can cause you to bleed too much if you don't stop taking them before surgery. Depending on the type of drug and the dose, your doctor will advise you to stop taking certain drugs or perhaps adjust your dosage a few weeks to a few days before your operation.

Ask about substitute medications and supplements. Your doctor may also recommend substitute medications of another type to help you control your pain in the mean time. As noted earlier, you can continue to take disease-modifying drugs like methotrexate and prednisone (common drugs for treating rheumatoid arthritis) until the day of your operation. Be sure to review with your doctor all of the medications, including those for other medical conditions such as heart disease, as well as any supplements you may be taking.

Consider blood donation. If you are having major surgery such as joint replacement, talk to your doctor about **autologous** (reinfusing blood from your own body) and **directed** (transfusing blood from one person to another) blood donation. In some cases hip and knee replacement can cause you to lose enough blood that you'll need a transfusion. The safest type of transfusion uses your own blood, which you can donate in advance of your operation. If you decide to do this, consult your doctor about an appropriate donation schedule. There are new blood donation techniques that allow you to reuse your own blood during or just after surgery. These are called intraoperative salvage (where a machine, called a cell saver, collects lost blood and processes it for re-use) and post-operative cell salvage (where collected blood is transfused after your surgery is done). If you can't donate your own blood, your family members and friends with the same blood type can donate blood for you in directed donation. If this is not an option, then the hospital can use blood from a blood bank.

Organize your medical information. Put together all of your medical information in one convenient file. This information should include: the names and contact information for the doctors you see; your medical conditions and the medications and supplements you take; any allergies you have to medications or anesthesia; your insurance coverage and the contact number plus any authorization numbers that may be required for surgery or a hospital stay; any dietary restrictions you have; legal information such as power of attorney or a living will. Make sure that a family member or close friend has access to this information in case it is needed while you are undergoing surgery or are in recovery.

Prepare your home. Because your ability to get around will be fairly limited right after surgery, you'll want to prepare your home in advance for your return. Talk with your doctor about what you'll be able to do, and make your home as comfortable and convenient as possible for your recovery. Make sure a friend or family member is available to stay with you initially to help out. If not, arrange for a nurse or home health aid for the first few days or week.

After hip or knee surgery, you won't be able to climb stairs at first, so arrange a comfortable recovery room on the first floor of your home. Arrange a place to sleep, such as an extra bedroom or foldout sofa, and place items you'll need nearby. Include a table for books and magazines, perhaps a television and telephone, medication, and a pitcher and glass. Remove throw rugs, electrical cords and anything else that could make you trip easily. Clear pathways throughout the house to make it as easy as possible for you to get around using crutches or a walker.

Stock your kitchen with easy or ready-made meals and snacks that won't require too much effort to prepare. You'll also want to put items in the kitchen and throughout the house within easy reach at arm's level so you won't have trouble getting what you need.

Obtain any assistive items that can make things easier for you right after surgery. These will probably include a walker, and perhaps crutches, bathroom grab bars, a bath seat, a three-in-one commode seat (which includes a bedside commode, raised toilet seat and shower seat), long-handled reachers, sock-pulling aids or shoe horns, a hand-held shower head attachment, and possibly a temporary handicapped parking permit. Other than the temporary handicapped parking permit (your doctor can authorize this, but you would get one from your local Department of Motor Vehicles), most of this equipment usually is given to you while you are in the hospital, or arranged through a hospital case manager to be delivered to your home through a medical-supply store or company.

Make other medical preparations. To help prevent possible complications, arrange any dental work or teeth cleaning that you need done well before your joint surgery. Remember, even minor infections anywhere in your body could travel to the surgery site and cause serious problems. Notify your surgeon if you come down with a cold or any other infection close to your surgery date. That will need to be cleared up before your operation.

In addition, you should have a pre-surgery exam and have some medical tests before your operation. These are routine procedures that may include having blood work done, providing a urine sample, and having a cardiogram and X-rays taken. You should also meet with the hospital's anesthesiologist to go over your anesthesia options. Together with your surgeon, you will make a decision about what type of anesthesia to have during your upcoming procedure. (See page 114.)

continued on p. 127

Preparing Your Home for After Surgery: Seven Handy Tips

When you first come home from the hospital after your surgery, you won't be able to spring back into your normal routine. In fact, you may find it very difficult just to get around the house and to do your normal activities. You won't be able to walk up and down stairs, and you may need assistance from others to do your basic bathing, dressing and grooming, or to prepare meals.

Preparing your home in advance for your return from the hospital will make your transition much easier. Here are some easy strategies for doing so:

1. Discuss what movements or tasks you will be able to do, and what you will not be able to do, with your doctor. He or his assistants may have some guidelines for you to make your home as comfortable and convenient as possible for your recovery.

2. Make advance arrangements for one of your family members or a friend to accompany you home from the hospital and to stay with you initially to help out. If you don't have anyone who can fill this role, make advance arrangements for a home-care nurse or similar hired professional help for the first few days or week of your recovery. Discuss fees well in advance, and see if your insurance will cover this cost.

3. Climbing stairs may not be possible during the early part of your recovery. So if you normally sleep on the second floor of your home (or downstairs in a basement room), arrange a comfortable recovery room on the first floor of your home. Have some-

one help you set up a place to sleep, either by moving a bed or foldout sofa bed into the living area, or moving your necessary items into an extra bedroom.

Place items you'll need nearby and within easy reach from your bed. If there is no nightstand next to your bed, either move one into your temporary sleeping area up a temporary table with a light and essential items. Put books and magazines within your reach, medication, tissues, a pitcher of water, and a cup or glass. If possible, hook up a telephone receiver (or portable unit) and TV in your temporary sleeping area for your comfort and convenience.

4. Falls can be very dangerous when you have just had joint surgery. So you will want to modify and clear your home's pathways to reduce the chance of slips and falls, and make it as easy as possible for you to get around using crutches or a walker.

   Remove any throw rugs, tack down any loose carpeting, rearrange any electrical cords that you could trip over, and move anything else, such as a potted plant or magazine rack, that you easily could trip over.

5. Cooking and preparing meals can be very tiring and difficult during your early recovery from surgery. So plan ahead if you don't have someone who can stay with you and prepare all your meals for you. Stock your refrigerator or freezer with ready-made meals and snacks that won't require too much effort to prepare. Put any kitchen scissors or bag clips within easy reach in case you need to open or seal a bagged item.

Preparing Your Home for After Surgery: Seven Handy Tips *(cont.)*

Put anything – drinking cups, paper towels or resealable bags – in the kitchen and throughout the house in an accessible place (such as on your kitchen counter), at arm's level so you won't have trouble reaching them when you need them.

6. Gather some assistive devices to help you with your recovery. Assistive devices are instruments designed to help you move around, do normal activities and access necessary items easier, particularly when you are recovering from surgery and have limited ability to bend, stoop, walk or reach.

   Assistive devices include a walker or crutches, bathroom grab bars, a raised toilet seat attachment, a temporary ramp, drawer or door pulls, rotating attachments that help you get in and out of a car, long-handled reachers and grippers, dressing aids and shoehorns.

   For more information about making your home more "joint-friendly" and using assistive devices, read *Tips for Good Living With Arthritis,* a book from the Arthritis Foundation. This handy guide is filled with more than 700 tips for making ordinary activities easier on joints and muscles, and how to adapt your home and lifestyle for easier use all around. Order *Tips* for only $9.95 (plus shipping and handling) by calling 800/207-8633 or logging on to www.arthritis.org.

7. Ask your doctor to issue you a temporary handicapped-parking permit for your car. Although you may not be driving right away, your driver can park closer to entrances of doctor's offices, stores and other places you need to go.

JUST BEFORE SURGERY

While you will be making many of your surgery preparations well in advance, there are a few things you'll need to do in the last couple of days before your operation. You'll need to pack a small suitcase for the hospital containing some comfortable, loose-fitting clothes, toiletries, and non-skid slippers or shoes (preferably slip-on).

Also take copies of your insurance cards, a picture ID, medications you regularly take, and a magazine or other reading material. Be sure to leave any jewelry, valuables and your wallet at home, though you may want to take a small amount of cash for newspapers, etc., during your hospital stay. Entrust anything else to your family member or friend who accompanies you to the hospital.

Make sure the hospital has notified you of your admission time by the day before your surgery at the latest. If not, contact the hospital. Take a shower or bath the day before your surgery, since you will have a tough time bathing right after the operation. Don't eat or drink anything after midnight the night before, so your stomach will be empty to prevent nausea associated with the anesthesia. And get a good night's sleep.

QUESTIONS TO ASK BEFORE SURGERY

Here are some questions to ask before your operation takes place:

- How long will the surgery take?
- How long will I be in the recovery room?
- Does the hospital and doctor have all of your medical information and any hospitalization confirmation numbers from your insurance company?
- What should I bring to the hospital? (See page 128 for suggestions.)
- When can family members see me after the surgery?

What To Pack

Make sure you have these essential items for your hospital stay:
- Comfortable, loose-fitting clothes, such as sweats or shorts
- Toiletry items (only the essentials – the hospital is not a beauty contest)
- Non-skid slippers or shoes (preferably slip-on)
- Insurance cards
- Identification card with photograph (such as your driver's license)
- Any medications you regularly take
- Magazines, books or other reading material
- A small amount of cash for newspapers or snacks, in a small change purse

Don't take:
- Jewelry or even a nice watch
- Valuables of any kind
- Your wallet

Entrust anything else to your family member or friend who accompanies you to the hospital. Unfortunately, people staying in hospitals often have their valuables stolen. Don't take that chance! You will have enough things on your plate – you don't need to have to deal with getting a new driver's license or credit cards in addition to your recovery.

- Do I need physical therapy before the operation? When will it begin after the surgery?
- What are the possible complications of surgery? What are the surgeon's plans to handle any complications that may arise?
- How soon will I go home from the hospital after surgery?
- What pain-relief options will be available to me after surgery?

PHYSICAL THERAPY

Physical therapy focuses on using your joints and muscles to the best of your ability to help you regain or improve how your body functions. If you have pain or a limiting condition like arthritis, physical therapy can help you to maximize your abilities by strengthening your muscles and joints. Physical therapy is also part of rehabilitation from surgery. A physical therapist is a health professional with specialized training in developing specialized exercise plans and other techniques to help patients improve their ability to function after illness, injury or surgery.

In some cases you may see a physical therapist before your operation. He or she may educate you about the exercises and activities you'll need to do after surgery to aid your recovery. In addition, if you are having trouble exercising as you prepare for surgery, a physical therapist can offer a customized plan and some modifications to make exercise possible for you.

Physical therapy plays an important role in your recovery after surgery. You're likely to see a physical therapist very soon – perhaps the first day – after your operation to begin exercises to help you recover. The hospital will likely assign a physical therapist to you while you are in the hospital. Your surgeon might recommend or refer you to an outside physical therapist for post-surgical rehabilitation should you need it.

Take Control of Your Health

You may think that joint surgery only involves you, your surgeon and the hospital nurses. But, in fact, a whole team of health professionals is involved in your operation. Of course that team will include you, your doctor, your surgeon and the hospital nurses. In addition to those, others who play a role on your health care team include: an anesthesiologist, physical therapist, perhaps an occupational therapist, and any rehabilitation facility staff, home health aids or nurses you have help you at home.

All of these health professionals have specific jobs to do in taking care of you during your joint surgery. Some are involved in the operation itself, while others help you through your recovery. While each of these health professionals has a specific area of expertise, they must also be a part of the overall team involved in your care. And you have a job to do as well. Your role is to be a sort of coach to this health care team. You'll need to communicate with each of them and make sure that they communicate with each other during the process of your joint surgery and recovery.

Although the health professionals are experts in their specific areas, you are the expert on you. Make sure that you get what you need and have your questions answered if you don't understand something. You are the manager of your own health, and each of the health professionals on your team is there to advise you and help you to do the best job of managing your own health. You should be completely informed about your operation and everything that happens to you along the way. Be sure you take the opportunity to be the coach of your health care team and take an active role, rather than a passive one, in your own health care.

Typically there is a plan of specific capabilities you'll need to achieve and activities you'll need to be able to do before you are discharged from the hospital. A physical therapist will help you with a plan to accomplish these goals and to regain your strength after the operation. In addition, you will likely attend physical therapy appointments after you leave the hospital to help you continue your progress through recovery.

chapter 7:

Tips for Losing Weight Before Surgery

Being overweight can complicate joint surgery because it makes the job more difficult for your surgeon. Excess weight makes it harder for the surgeon to be precise in his work and to gain access to the parts of the body he needs to reach. Extra pounds can also make the recovery more difficult for you by putting more weight on fragile new joints and on weakened muscles.

If you are overweight and considering joint surgery, your doctor may recommend losing some weight before the operation. In some cases, a surgeon may refuse to operate until a patient loses weight because of the risk of complications during surgery.

The good news is that losing weight will not only improve the outcome of your operation, but it will also be good for your health in general. Excess weight is already a contributing factor to osteoarthritis, meaning that being overweight can actually help cause the development of the disease.

Additional pounds of weight on your body increase the amount of pressure that joints such as your knees and hips must support. The additional weight also increases the amount of pressure and impact that these joints must absorb with each step that you take.

For example, for every extra pound of body weight, your knees gain three pounds of added stress. For your hips, this same amount of additional weight translates to six times the amount of pressure. Losing weight will remove extra stress and pressure from your joints, including those that aren't yet painful enough to require surgery.

In the long run, losing weight and keeping it off could help you avoid surgery on other joints in the future. Plus, the need for losing weight in order to have surgery can be a good incentive to keep you motivated.

The Lowdown on Weight Loss

While we all wish there were an easy plan, a simple pill or some other quick fix to help us lose weight fast, the truth is that there is no magic bullet for weight loss. The only effective way to lose weight is to burn more calories than you consume. And the best way to do that is by increasing your activity level and reducing the amount of calories you eat.

The best way to lose weight is to change your overall habits and lose weight gradually as you stick with an overall healthy lifestyle. If your goal is to lose weight for surgery, you may need to work on your weight-loss plan and then schedule your operation once you've made progress. Weight loss takes a while. Trying to lose weight with a specific date in mind can be stressful, and you may not be able to achieve the deadline. Talk with your doctor and surgeon about an effective plan. Perhaps you can spend a few months following a healthful plan and then reassess your surgery plan.

Don't try to lose a lot of weight quickly in just a few weeks. Some fads can help you lose weight quickly at first, but once you stop the dieting you can put on the pounds again rapidly, plus some.

With any weight-loss plan, you should talk to your doctor first for advice and precautions. You may need to make sure that when you reduce your calorie intake you still get enough of certain vitamins and nutrients that you need to be healthy. Your doctor can also give you recommendations on safe forms of exercise you can do without harming your joints. You may want to see a nutritionist or registered dietitian, too, for help with designing and maintaining a healthful eating plan.

The Basic Pillars of a Healthy Diet

The basic pillars of a healthy diet can give you a general framework for the diet portion of your weight-loss plan. These guidelines are:

1. Eat a variety of foods that follow the guidelines of your physician, dietitian or the USDA Food Guide Pyramid (see the section on this model on page 136).
2. Consume only moderate amounts of fat and cholesterol.
3. Include lots of vegetables, fruits and grains.
4. Eat only moderate amounts of sugar.
5. Drink alcohol only in moderation, if at all. (If you are taking any medications for your pain or inflammation, drinking alcohol may be dangerous to your health. Ask your physician.)
6. Limit your use of salt.
7. Drink eight glasses of water each day.

Here's how these strategies help you lose weight and develop a nutritionally balanced diet. Eating a variety of foods from several groups, such as dairy, meat and vegetables, helps your body get the many nutrients it needs to be healthy. Fruits and vegetables, in particular, are important sources of many vitamins and minerals your body needs, as well as of **antioxidants** and other plant chemicals that help fight disease.

Antioxidants are important chemicals that help neutralize substances called **free radicals** in the body. These free radicals can cause damage to the body if allowed to float free, but antioxidants help to neutralize these damaging effects. Common antioxidants include vitamins C and E and beta carotene. These are typically found in fresh fruits and vegetables, such as broccoli, red peppers, citrus fruits, blueberries, as well as vegetable oils, eggs and whole-grain cereals.

By moderating fat, cholesterol and sugar in your diet, you reduce some of the highest calorie foods. Some of these foods include cookies, cakes, sweets, fried foods, meat, potato chips and snack foods, prepackaged foods and alcohol. In order to lose weight you have to use more calories than you consume, so lowering the amount of calories you consume can help you work toward this goal. This can help cut your calorie intake right away. Plus, reducing fat and cholesterol is good for your heart. Alcohol is another high-calorie indulgence, so if you do drink, do so in moderation to help lower the amount of calories you consume.

Limiting your use of salt is a general guideline for healthful eating, and it can be especially important for people with certain medical conditions such as high blood pressure. Excess salt intake has been linked to higher blood pressure (a condition also known as **hypertension**) in some studies, and doctors generally discourage consuming more than three grams of salt per day.

Be careful to take note of salt (or sodium) in the many foods you eat – salt is not just the table salt you may shake on your baked potato or lamb chops. Read the nutrition labels on packaged foods to see how much sodium the food contains. Packaged or processed foods, including frozen meals and canned soups, may have excessive amounts of salt as a preservative or flavoring. Most supermarkets will carry brands of packaged foods that have lower amounts of salt or sodium. Use dried herbs or salt substitute mixes instead of table salt to flavor your foods. You may find this seasoning to be a tasty alternative!

Finally, drinking eight glasses of water per day helps your body to run efficiently and remove waste effectively. In addition, drinking plenty of water will help you to feel full so that you eat less, particularly if you drink water before a meal.

THE FOOD GUIDE PYRAMID

The U.S. Department of Agriculture has designed the Food Guide Pyramid to assist you in devising a healthful eating plan. Use this pyramid as a guide to preparing meals and assessing what you're eating each day. The pyramid recommends following a diet that contains more of the foods at the base of the pyramid, such as whole grains, fruits and vegetables and smaller amounts of foods higher on the pyramid, such as meat, dairy foods and sweets.

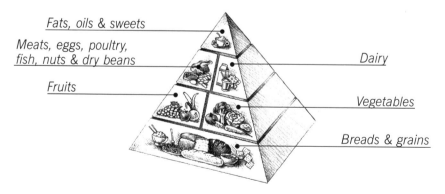

The USDA Food Guide Pyramid

TIPS FOR READING FOOD LABELS

One way you can take control of how much fat, cholesterol and calories you consume is by reading your food labels. These labels not only include a list of ingredients in the food, but also a standardized account of the nutritional content, including fat, cholesterol, calories, protein, carbohydrates, sodium, sugar, fiber and vitamins. The labels allow you to compare the content of different foods.

In addition, the government has set criteria for labeling foods "low-fat," "fat-free," "reduced-fat," "low-sodium" and other terms you see on packaging at the grocery store and in food advertising. These terms can confuse people who are trying to create a healthy diet. Remember, eating foods that are low fat or even nonfat does not mean you can eat as much as you want without damaging your diet. These foods often have plenty of calories, even an excess of calories due to their high sugar content.

Here is a thumbnail guide to food label claims:

- **"Light"** – food contains 1/3 fewer calories or 1/2 the fat of the regular, reference version of the food
- **"Low"** – you can eat a large amount of the food without exceeding the daily value of the nutrient labeled "low"
- **"Fat-free"** – naturally contains no fat; indicates that the food has less than .5 g of fat per serving
- **"High"** – contains 20 percent or more of the daily value for the nutrient in one serving

Monitoring your food labels more carefully can help you avoid too much fat, cholesterol, sugar and sodium in your meals. Become a master of reading food labels. You will not only realize that some of your regular grocery purchases have undesirable amounts of these nutrients. You will also discover some great foods for meals and snacks that are healthy and taste great too.

CONTROLLING PORTION SIZES

Another important way you can monitor what you eat to lose weight is to take control of the portions you eat. Especially at restaurants, you can easily eat much more of a particular food than you need for a healthful meal. Many restaurants try to provide value for their customers, value which translates to large portions of food – much more than you would ordinarily eat at home. And even at home, you may be unaware of what constitutes a proper portion of various foods, which can mean you're eating more calories and fat than you need.

food group	serving size	visual comparison
GRAINS	1 slice of bread 1/2 cup of cooked cereal, rice or pasta 1 ounce of ready-to-eat cereal	2 tablespoons of peanut butter 1/2 cup cooked pasta (scoop of ice cream)
VEGETABLES	1/2 cup of chopped raw or cooked veggies 1 cup of leafy raw veggies	1 cup dry cereal (large handful)
FRUITS	1 medium apple, orange or banana 1/2 cup of juice 1/2 cup of canned fruit 1/2 cup of dried fruit	1 cup of veggies (your fist) medium piece of fruit (a baseball)
DAIRY	1 cup of milk or yogurt 2 ounces of cheese	2 ounces of cheese (a pair of dominoes)
PROTEIN FOODS	3 ounces of cooked lean meat, poultry or fish 1/2 cup of cooked dry beans 1 egg counts as 1 ounce of lean meat	3 ounces of meat or fish (palm of your hand) 1 teaspoon of butter (the tip of your thumb)

By taking control of portion sizes, you can make sure you eat less fat and fewer calories in order to lose weight. Here are some tricks to help you assess a proper portion size:

It may be useful for you to purchase a kitchen food scale, a set of nested dry measuring cups, measuring spoons and a liquid measuring cup. These tools will help you accurately measure portions of foods you prepare at home. After a while, you will become accustomed to how large the right portion looks, and you may not have to use the measuring tools often.

These tools may be found at most supermarkets, discount department stores, hardware stores and cooking supply stores. Cooking supply stores may also carry miniature food scales that you can take to restaurants, if you choose. If measuring your portions in restaurants is not your style, use the visual guidelines on page 138 or check menus for weights of items like meat or fish.

EXERCISE AND ACTIVITY

The other half of any weight-loss plan is exercise and activity. In addition to eating fewer calories and less fat, you also need to use up the energy you consume in food. That means moving around as much as possible.

If you have been inactive or have pain in a particular joint (such as the one being considered for surgery), be sure to talk with your doctor first about the proper type of exercise for you. In addition, choose something you feel comfortable with and that you like, so that you're more likely to enjoy it and to stick with it. The type of exercise you choose should also been convenient so that you are able to do it regularly.

Along with exercising on a regular basis, you can add activity to your daily routine in a number of ways that can help you burn calories. Try taking the stairs instead of the elevator and parking further away when you

Calorie Burning Chart

The following chart can help you figure out how many calories are burned during certain activities. These figures show the amount of calories burned per hour of activity for a 150-lb. person.

Activity	Calories
Bicycling	210
Calisthenics	310
Dance	340
Hiking	300
Jogging	650
Swimming (fast)	630
Swimming (slow)	320
Tennis	420
Walking	210

go to the store. Take a lap around the mall before you start shopping. Push your grocery cart through aisles first before you start filling it. Think of other creative ways you can add movement throughout your day.

LOOKING AHEAD

In the next chapter, we'll look at some ways to use exercise to prepare your body for a successful surgery and recovery.

A metal component is attached to the end of the femur using bone cement

A plastic component is cemented to the back of the patella

A plastic plate is attached to the metal tibia component

A metal component is secured to the end of the tibia

cement?

Pelvis

A special plastic liner is
locked into the metal shell

A metal implant
is placed into
the hollowed
femur

A metal ball
attached to
metal impla

The damaged ball is cut off of
the femur bone.

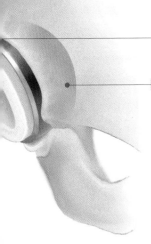

Pelvis

A metal shell is pressed
into the hip socket

Bone graft material

component is
he stem of the
ht

Hip Joint After Surgery

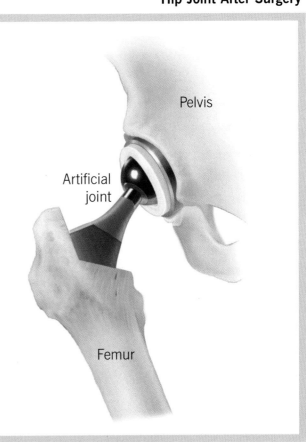

Pelvis

Artificial
joint

Femur

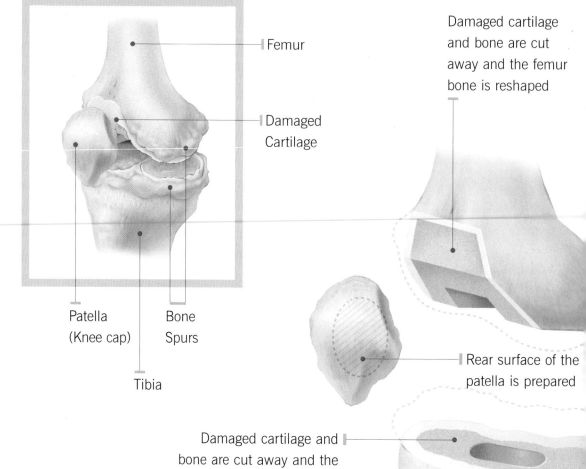

Femur

Damaged
Cartilage

Patella
(Knee cap)

Bone
Spurs

Tibia

Damaged cartilage
and bone are cut
away and the femur
bone is reshaped

Rear surface of the
patella is prepared

Damaged cartilage and
bone are cut away and the
tibia bone is reshaped

Joint After Surgery

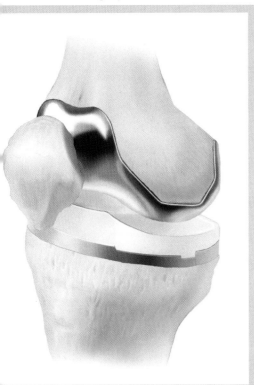

Unicondylar Knee Replacement

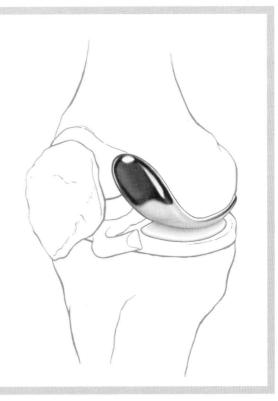

– OR –

Unicondylar Knee Replacement
Unlike total knee replacement surgery, this less invasive procedure replaces only the damaged or arthritic parts of the knee.

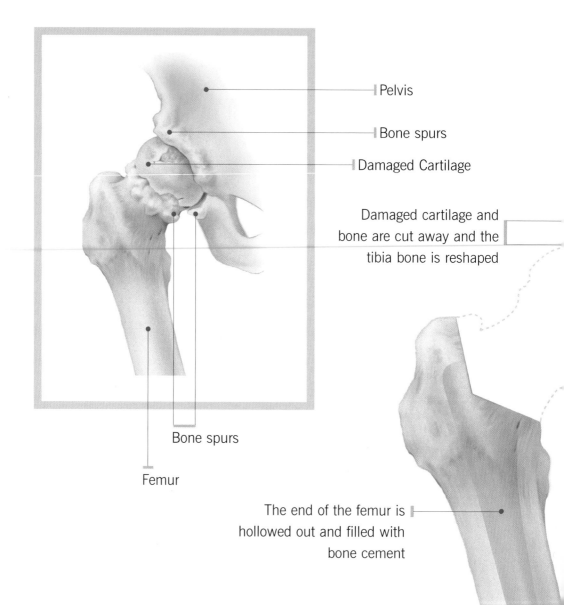

Pelvis

Bone spurs

Damaged Cartilage

Damaged cartilage and bone are cut away and the tibia bone is reshaped

Bone spurs

Femur

The end of the femur is hollowed out and filled with bone cement

chapter 8:

Exercise Before Surgery

Recovery from joint surgery is a challenge for anybody. But you can make it easier on yourself by preparing ahead of time. After surgery, your mobility will be limited for a while and your muscles will need time to heal from the operation. This means they will need to regain strength and stability gradually.

One way to make your recovery quicker and smoother is to be in the best shape you can be before you have surgery. In addition to losing weight if you need to, you can also exercise to build strength in your muscles so they have a head start for your recovery. This is also important for your muscles that won't be directly affected by the operation. Until you regain strength in your new joint, the muscles of your other side will have extra work to do in supporting your body. If you can't bear weight on the leg that was operated on until it heals, you'll have to compensate by putting additional weight on the other leg to help hold you up. Building strength in them beforehand will ensure that they're prepared to handle the job.

Your recovery will also include exercises you must do to help your body heal and strengthen. Your physical therapist will guide you in a recovery exercise routine that suits your surgery and your needs. You will be building strength in your muscles and working your new (or surgically repaired) joint to increase flexibility and range of motion.

Ways To Get in Shape Before Your Surgery

There are a number of ways to get in better physical shape before your surgery. We have offered a few easy ideas for you to consider and discuss with your surgeon. You and your doctor know your limitations and exercise-related hurdles, both physical and mental. So finding the right course of action to get in shape before your operation is important. Talk openly to your doctor.

Because you'll have many other challenges to think about, you may find it helpful to become familiar with these exercises before your operation. Talk to your doctor or physical therapist for instructions on these exercises so you can learn them in advance. Some of them may be very similar to the ones we'll show here, depending on what type of surgery you have.

WALKING

If you are having hip or knee surgery, your leg muscles will need to be strong. Inactivity and the effects of surgery will weaken your muscles right after your operation. Plus your muscles will have to provide extra support as your joint heals. Having these muscles as strong as possible to begin with will help with both of these situations.

A walking program focuses on the large muscles of your legs. This program will help strengthen these important muscles. Even if you have trouble doing other types of exercise because of pain, you can probably do some amount of walking. Walking is also a great way to incorporate cardiovascular exercise into your fitness routine. This type of exercise raises your heart rate and helps you burn calories and keep your cardiovascular (heart, arteries and veins) system in good shape.

Walking can be done anytime and any place, so it is convenient and easy to adapt. If you have trouble walking for long distances at one time, you can add shorter stints of walking into your routine throughout the day. Building your muscles through walking can help prepare you for your recovery after surgery.

The Arthritis Foundation publishes an excellent guide on walking that can be used by anyone with joint problems or pain. *Walk With Ease: Your Guide to Walking for Better Health, Improved Fitness and Less Pain* is $11.95 and may be purchased by calling 800/207-8633 or logging on to www.arthritis.org.

BICYCLING

Bicycling is another adaptable, cardiovascular and strength-building exercise you can do at your own pace. In addition, it is generally relatively gentle on your joints. Plus, bicycling is a good activity for strengthening your leg muscles, especially the quadriceps muscles in your thighs. It is also an exercise that generally is comfortable for people with knee pain to do. Bicycling options include riding a bike around your neighborhood streets, or riding a stationary bike at home or in the gym.

Strengthening Exercises

The following exercises target the large muscle groups of your legs to help strengthen them. As with any type of exercise, check with your doctor first to make sure the exercises are appropriate for you.

1. Back Kick

Rest your hands on a chair for balance and stand straight on one leg. Lift the other leg behind you. Hold for three seconds. Try to keep your leg straight as you move it backward. Move only your hip and leg, not your waist. Keep your upper body straight. You can add resistance to this exercise by using an elastic exercise band around your ankles. Repeat the exercise with the other leg.

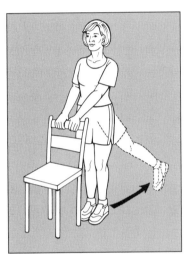

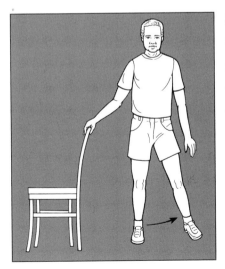

2. Side Leg Kick

Stand near a chair and hold it for support. Stand on one leg and lift the other leg out to the side. Hold for three seconds then lower the leg. Don't lean toward the chair. Repeat with the other leg. Resistance can be added with an elastic exercise band.

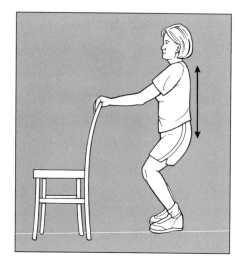

3. Skier's Squat

Stand behind a chair with your hands lightly resting on the top of it for support. Keep your feet flat on the floor. Keep your back straight and slowly bend your knees to lower your body a few inches. Hold for three to six seconds, then slowly raise back up.

4. Thigh Firmer and Knee Stretch

Sit on the edge of a chair or lie on your back with your legs stretched out in front and your heels resting on the floor. Tighten the muscle that runs across the front of the knee by pulling your toes toward your head. Push the back of the knee down toward the floor so that you also feel a

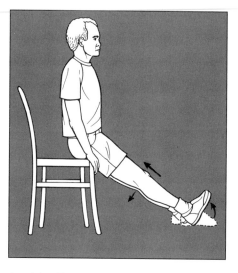

stretch at the back of your knee and ankle. For a greater stretch, put your heel on a footstool and lean forward as you pull your toes toward your head. Repeat with the other leg.

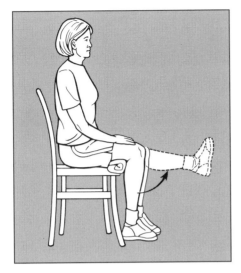

5. Knee Extension

Sit in a chair with your feet shoulder-width apart, and your knees directly above them. Put a towel under your knees for padding. With your hands on your thighs, raise your right leg to the count of three until your knee is straight but not locked. Pause, then lower your leg to the count of three. Repeat on the left side.

6. Calf Stretch

Stand behind a chair and hold the top of it lightly for support. Bend the knee of the leg you are not stretching so that it almost touches the chair. Put the leg to be stretched behind you, keeping both feet flat on the floor. Lean forward gently, keeping your back knee straight. Switch legs and repeat to stretch the other side.

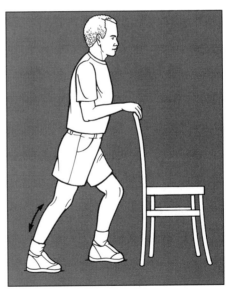

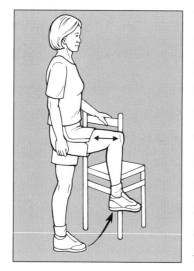

7. Knee Raises

Hold onto the back of a chair for support. Raise your knee toward your chest until your thigh is parallel to the floor. Lower your leg back to the floor, then repeat with your other leg. (Note: After most knee surgeries, you should not lift your knee so that it creates an angle greater than 90 degrees unless cleared by your doctor. Practice this technique now.)

HOW HEALTH-CARE PROFESSIONALS CAN HELP

If you have trouble staying motivated on your own to lose weight, or if you feel you need specific professional advice on diet and exercise, you can consult health professionals to help you with your goals.

Nutritionists and **dietitians** are professionals who have specialized education and training in diet and guiding others in creating, implementing and maintaining a healthful, personalized eating plan for optimum health. Nutritionists and dietitians can provide consultation on healthful eating habits, and often can provide an eating plan specifically geared toward your needs and goals. They can help you understand your eating habits and work toward changing them, and they can provide support and progress reports as you go.

These health-care professionals can also help ensure that you are getting the proper nutrients you need to stay healthy as you lose weight. Check with your doctor for a referral to a nutritionist or dietitian.

For help with an exercise plan, you can consult a physical therapist or **personal trainer**. Be sure to work with someone who has experience working with people who have joint problems like yours. You want to avoid someone who may recommend workouts that could be too strenuous or damaging to your joints. Ask your doctor's office for a referral, and be sure to check the credentials of any exercise specialist you engage. Make sure the person understands your health conditions and that you are about to have joint surgery.

Either of these professionals can help design an exercise program that meets your needs and that will help you reach your goals. They can also work with you to make sure you are performing exercises correctly to avoid injury, and they can help you stay motivated to follow your program.

LOOKING AHEAD

In this chapter, we've looked at how you can prepare physically by getting your body in shape to withstand the stress of surgery and recovery, including strength and flexibility.

Next, we'll see what you can expect from the operation itself so you feel you understand what will be happening to you during surgery. This information should help you feel more at ease with the procedure you are about to undergo. Knowing what to expect may help alleviate your fears or concerns, and allow you to go into your surgery with greater confidence and peace of mind.

chapter 9:

What Happens During Surgery

Now we come to one of the most mysterious parts of discussing surgery for patients: what takes place during the operation itself. In this chapter, we'll go over the surgical process step-by-step, from start to finish. Many of the steps are likely to be the same for different joint surgeries, while others will vary depending on the joint and type of operation. We'll spell out the differences for you here. This chapter will go over what to expect in the hospital. A special, full-color, illustrated foldout shows you the steps of the two most common surgeries: hip and knee replacement.

What You May Expect

Before you head to the hospital for your operation, you should have worked toward preparing yourself mentally and emotionally, as well as physically, for your surgery. The process of joint surgery is serious and challenging, so you should make sure that you are well prepared to handle everything you will experience. In addition, as you go into surgery, it is important to gear yourself up mentally. Approach the operation with a positive attitude and set yourself up mentally to take on the physical and emotional challenges and get through them.

You should also have your support network of family and friends on call and ready to help out. Make sure that everyone knows when the operation will take place and when you anticipate coming home. Ensure that those you've enlisted to help with getting to and from the hospital know when and where you need them to be. You'll need emotional as well as physical support as you go through the surgery and recover process. Be sure that you have your support network lined up to do what you need before you go to the hospital for your operation. You won't have the energy to round people up to help you after your operation.

At this point, you also should have made any necessary preparations at home for your return. As we discussed in Chapter 6, be sure that your refrigerator is stocked and that your recuperation area is set up before you head to the hospital. You also should have made all necessary arrangements for your check-in at the hospital, including any paperwork and pre-surgery laboratory tests. Before surgery, you should have had a pre-surgery medical exam, provided blood and urine samples to check for infections, X-rays and possibly a cardiogram.

As we discussed in Chapter 6, you will pack a small suitcase or duffel bag with the essential personal items for your hospital stay.

Again, you should also take with you your insurance card and any pre-admittance paperwork you're your doctor has told you will need to present when you check in. You may want to have a small amount of cash with you, as well, for incidental expenses like sodas or reading material. Take any medications that you use regularly and that your doctor has approved for you to take up until your operation and afterward. Again, leave any jewelry, credit cards or valuables at home or with a friend. You won't want to worry about keeping track of these items or of losing them. You won't need them during surgery. They can be stolen or lost easily while you are not in your room.

HOSPITAL ARRIVAL AND CHECK-IN

When you arrive at the hospital you'll have to check in at the admissions desk. Here, a staff member will go over your admission paperwork with you to make sure everything is in order. You'll need your identification and insurance card. Then you will change into a hospital gown, receive a hospital identification bracelet, and have your temperature, blood pressure and pulse checked. Your personal belongings will be stored safely. This process may take about an hour.

PRE-OPERATION

At this point, your family members will have to leave you so that you can be prepared for surgery. Here, your laboratory test results will be double-checked and you'll receive intravenous lines, narrow flexible tubes inserted into your veins to allow fluids or medications into your body. The anesthesiologist probably will check in with you at this point to confirm your choice of anesthesia (See the section in Chapter 6 on anesthesia).

Surgery (1-3 hours)

Next, you will receive anesthesia, either through an **intravenous** line (IV) or through a tube inserted in your back if you have chosen spinal or epidural anesthesia. A catheter, the long, thin, flexible tube that allows liquid to flow into or out of your body, will be attached to your bladder to eliminate waste during surgery.

You will be wearing your hospital gown and may be covered with a sheet. You'll be lying down on a wheeled table until you are taken into the operating room. Nurses will be monitoring you as the anesthesia takes effect. Once in the operating room, you'll be positioned properly for the type of surgery you'll be having (see below). The surgical staff will take you into the operating room and the operation will begin.

HIP REPLACEMENT

For hip replacement surgery, you will be placed on your side, with the hip to be operated on facing upward. Because you will have to stay in that position for a couple of hours, special supports will help hold you in place.

Next, the surgeon will make an **incision**, or a surgical cut of about six to 12 inches along your hip. Then he will separate the thighbone from the socket of the hip joint. Next he'll remove the head of the femur, or the rounded ball portion of your thighbone, using a special power bone saw. (Don't worry – this won't be the power saw you use to do woodworking at home, but a sanitary, oscillating small saw that is designed specifically for surgery.) The surgeon will use a tool called a reamer, which is a cutting tool with a rotating blade, to remove damaged bone and cartilage from the joint socket. Bone is cut away in very small amounts.

The surgeon will then fit the **acetabulum** component of the hip implant into the socket. The acetabulum is the upper cup-like component of the joint implant, into which the rounded head of the femoral component will fit. It consists of a metal shell and an inner plastic liner for the cup. Next he will prepare the femur by removing some of the center of the bone to make room for the implant. The femoral component of the implant will be put in place, either by fitting it snugly into the bone or by using a special bone cement to secure it. (See the section in Chapter 4 on cemented vs. cementless joint implants.) Finally, your surgeon will attach any of the soft tissues like muscles and ligaments that were cut during the operation to help secure the joint components within your leg.

KNEE REPLACEMENT

For knee replacement, the surgeon will first make an incision of about six or seven inches in your knee. Then he'll remove the damaged sections of the femur and the cartilage in small amounts. The femur is reshaped slightly to prepare it for the implant. In knee surgery, specialized guides or cutting jigs are used to make sure the bone is cut for a precise fit with the new joint component.

Then, the metal portion of the implant is attached to the femur with bone cement. The majority of knee replacements are secured using bone cement. In a cementless implant, however, screws or pegs may be used to secure the implant in place until new bone grows to hold it. A cementless procedure is often called **press-fit**. In some cases, a combination of techniques is used so that the femoral component (which attaches to the thigh bone) does not use cement and the tibial component (which attaches to the shin bone) does use cement.

Next, the surgeon removes the damaged parts of the tibia, or shinbone, and cartilage and reshapes the bone to fit the implant. Then that portion of the implant is attached with bone cement. The surgeon attaches a plastic plate to the tibia portion of the implant.

Finally, a plastic component is attached to the back of the kneecap. This component is a small, round plastic piece about the size and shape of the kneecap bone, or patella. It is attached to the back of the kneecap with bone cement (called methylmethacrylate) and allows the kneecap to move smoothly over the other new joint components. If the knee joint is replaced using a press-fit procedure, the bone will grow over the prosthesis over several months. Cemented implants are stable from the moment the procedure is done.

SHOULDER REPLACEMENT

The surgeon makes a three- to four-inch incision along your upper arm, from the collarbone to where the muscle attaches to the bone of the upper arm. He then cuts away the head of the humerus bone (upper arm) and uses reamers to create a cavity large enough in the bone for the implant. The metal stem is inserted into the bone and attached with bone cement. A metal head component is attached to the top of the humerus bone. Then he smoothes the socket of the shoulder joint to fit the shape of the new shoulder socket piece.

Next he attaches the glenoid, or shoulder socket, component of the implant with bone cement. Cementless versions are fitted tightly into the bone, and may temporarily be secured with pins or screws, until new bone grows into the implant to hold it in place. The tendons are then reattached.

To secure the joint after surgery, the limb is placed in a sling and a pillow is placed under the elbow for support.

Finger and Toe Joint Replacement

As in the other joint replacements, the surgeon makes an incision and removes the diseased or damaged portions of bone and cartilage from the joint. Then the artificial joint made of flexible material, such as silicone, and metal is implanted.

Unicondylar Knee Replacement

Unicondylar knee replacements are procedures used for patients affected by OA on only one side of their knee. The surgeon first makes an incision in your knee. Then he removes the damaged areas of cartilage and meniscus, a crescent-shaped piece of cartilage, from the knee. Next, the surgeon reshapes a portion of the tibia to prepare it for the implant. Then the plastic tibia component is attached with bone cement.

After that, the surgeon removes the damaged portion of the femur and reshapes it to fit the femoral component of the implant. Then he attaches the metal femur component with bone cement.

There are new, minimally invasive procedures used in some cases for this type of replacement. These procedures involve only a two-three-inch incision, and sometimes are performed on an outpatient basis. Ask your surgeon for more information on these procedures.

ARTHROSCOPY

In knee arthroscopy, the surgeon will make three small incisions in your knee. Through one incision, the surgeon will inject a sterile solution such as saline to expand the joint and provide a clear view within the knee. Then he will insert the arthroscope through another incision, and use a television screen to view the inside of your knee and assess the problem. These problems may include torn cartilage or a torn meniscus, a damaged ligament, loose pieces of bone or cartilage, or inflamed joint tissue.

Then, if necessary, he will insert a surgical instrument to cut away or otherwise treat damaged tissue, for example by trimming away a piece of torn cartilage or meniscus to ease pain, by reconstructing a torn ligament, removing inflamed joint tissue, or removing loose pieces of bone or cartilage.

ARTHRODESIS

Arthrodesis, or the fusion of a joint that is weak and unstable, is very uncommon in large joints such as the knee or hip, but is still used very successfully in smaller joints, such as the ankle, hand or foot. In arthrodesis, the ends of the bone are cut to fit together, and secured firmly together. The bones grow together just as a bone fracture would heal. The joint is fused, meaning that it will not have the mobility that it did when it was healthy, but will be stable.

OSTEOTOMY

In osteotomy, your surgeon will make an incision and then reshape the ends of the shinbone (tibia) or thighbone (femur) to improve these bones' alignment with your knee. He will then realign healthy bone and cartilage to compensate for the damaged tissue. He will reposition the joint, realigning the axis of the limb away from the area that is diseased or worn away. This technique lets your knee glide freely and carry your weight more evenly.

After the procedure, your doctor may use one of several techniques to hold your surgically repaired joint in place and keep the knee from moving around while it heals: a cast, staples or internal plate devices. Ask your surgeon which method he will use on your joint.

CLOSING

After the surgeon has completed the internal portion of your surgery, he will close your incision. For larger incisions, as in hip and knee replacement, the surgeon will use stitches, and for arthroscopy, with smaller incisions, he'll use either stitches or paper tape to hold the wound closed. Your general anesthesia, if you have chosen this option, will be stopped so that you gradually begin awakening as it wears off. You'll likely still feel a bit groggy for a while, but you'll gradually become more alert. Then you'll be taken to the anesthesia recovery room.

In the anesthesia recovery room, you'll likely be in a bed surrounded by a curtain to give you some privacy from other patients. Nurses will be checking on you periodically to monitor your recovery from the anesthesia. As you become more alert, the hospital staff may allow your family members to come in to see you.

If you've had arthroscopy, you'll go home from here once you've completely awakened. If you've had more involved surgery, you'll be transferred to your hospital room from here. You may have pillows placed underneath your knee to support it or between your knees to keep you from moving your legs together if you've had hip surgery.

What Is Going on While You're in Surgery?

During your operation, several members of your health-care team will be involved. These include the anesthesiologist, surgeon and probably several nurses. There may also be additional doctors assisting the surgeon.

They'll use a number of surgical instruments, such as a bone saw, reamer, scalpel and arthroscope, which is designed for specific tasks, such as making incisions or making it possible to reach the target joint. For knee replacement surgery, precise tools allow the surgeon to make accurate cuts in the bone when necessary and to help fit the implant in place accurately and securely. For hip replacement, a special, oscillating power saw is used to remove the head of the femur.

In addition, other instruments help monitor your **vital signs** such as blood pressure and heart rate during the operation. A catheter, or thin, flexible tube, inserted in your bladder will allow the elimination of waste during surgery. Most people cannot feel the catheter while it is inserted in the bladder. You may feel some slight discomfort during its removal, but this usually is relatively minor.

Generally, IVs should also be painless when they are in your arm and when they are removed. You may experience slight pain when they are inserted, and perhaps some slight bruising after they are removed. If you experience pain or swelling while the IV is inserted, however, notify a nurse because it may have to be removed.

COMMON QUESTIONS YOU MAY HAVE

You may be wondering some of the following things about your surgery:

Will it hurt? Because you'll receive anesthesia (either local or general), you should not feel pain during the operation. You will have some pain, though, after the operation once the anesthesia has worn off. We will go over post-operative pain control methods later in Chapter 10.

Should I watch? You will only have the option to observe your surgery if you have regional anesthesia. With general anesthesia, you'll be completely asleep during the whole thing. If you do have regional anesthesia, though, the decision of whether to watch is a personal one. To some people, it may be interesting and comforting to see what is going on. For others, though, seeing an operation on yourself may make you queasy and perhaps more nervous. Talk with your doctor as well as other people who have had the surgery to find out what they experienced before you decide.

How long will it take? A total hip replacement operation can take any-where from one to three hours to complete, while a knee replacement takes about two hours. Arthroscopic knee surgery usually takes about an hour to an hour and a half. You'll then spend an additional hour or two in the recovery room afterward. Minimally invasive knee replace-ment procedures may entail a shorter recovery period too. Discuss the expected length of your operation and recovery from anesthesia with your family so they will know what to expect.

IMMEDIATELY AFTER SURGERY

Right after your operation, you will be recovering mostly from the anes-thesia in the recovery room. You will continue to be monitored until you awaken. Nurses may place a pillow between your legs to keep them apart. You will stay in the anesthesia recovery room for about an hour or two. Once you wake up completely and you are stable, you will be moved to your hospital room.

Once in your room after the operation, you will receive medication for pain control, drugs known as analgesics. (See Chapter 3 for more information on these drugs.) Ask your doctor or nurse about the medication and side effects so you know what to expect.

If you had epidural anesthesia, you may still have the epidural attached in order to receive pain medication. If you had general anesthesia, you will have an intravenous line for pain medicine. The most common pain medications given intravenously after surgery are morphine and *Demerol*. In most cases, you can control the amount of pain medication you need up to the advisable limit. That way you can administer the medication as you need it. You will also likely receive **antibiotics** (usually *Cefazolin*) to prevent infection and blood-thinning medication to prevent blood clots.

Immediately after the operation, you may only be given ice chips and, a little later, a liquid diet. If you've had general anesthesia, the nurses will advise you to cough and breathe deeply to help clear your lungs. Fluid buildup in the lungs can be very dangerous, so it's important that you clear your lungs after surgery as directed by your nurses. Oral pain medications commonly prescribed after joint surgery include *Percocet, Vicodin, Lortab* and *Darvocet*.

If you've had knee surgery, you may have a drain attached to your knee to allow excess fluid to drain if it has built up around your knee. For both hip and knee surgery, you will be wearing elastic hose or special compression stockings or to help prevent blood clots in your legs.

Initially, you may feel nauseated and lose your appetite. You may receive laxatives and stool softeners to help ease constipation that can result from pain medication. Once the urinary catheter is removed after surgery, you may need to use a bedpan just at first until you can begin to move around and get to the bathroom. Your nurse will help you with the bedpan.

Some patients also experience difficulty sleeping after surgery that sometimes continues even at home. You will have some pain and discomfort until you're recovered completely, and this can make it hard to get comfortable and sleep well. Getting plenty of sound rest is important to your healing and recovery, so tell your doctor if you're having trouble sleeping. He can prescribe sleep medication for you. Common sleep medications include *Ambien, Halcion* and *Restoril.*

YOUR INITIAL RECOVERY

While you are still in the hospital, you will already be working on your overall recovery from surgery. In fact, there are several milestones you'll need to achieve in the hospital before your doctor will consider you to be ready to go home. These include getting in and out of bed, walking with crutches or a walker, moving your joint (such as bending and straightening your knee), climbing a few stairs, and being able to do your recovery exercises. Your hospital stay may last for three to seven days for total knee replacement and three to 10 days for total hip replacement.

First, it is important to begin moving your joints soon after surgery to regain your strength and promote healing. To help you begin to get movement back in your legs, your doctor may have you use a device that carefully moves your leg for you. This is called a **continuous passive motion machine** or CPM. The machine will gently bend and straighten your leg, and a nurse or physical therapist will set the machine to move a specified amount and speed. Your surgeon or therapist will prescribe certain movements for you. The machine keeps your leg elevated to reduce swelling and aids circulation in your leg.

In addition to the CPM machine, a physical therapist will come to see you in the hospital to begin your recovery exercises. You will work on exercises to rotate and pump your ankles to move blood through your legs. Plus there are other exercises you can do to move your knee or hip and regain strength in your large leg muscles.

In addition, you will begin to walk in the hospital, usually with the help of a walker or crutches. In your pre-surgery planning, find out whether the hospital will arrange for this equipment or whether you have to. Before your surgery, you should also explore what type of equipment your insurance policy will cover – either rental or purchase. A physical therapist can show you how to move properly with your crutches or walker.

Once you have achieved the necessary goals, and your doctor has confirmed that you are free of infection or other complications, you will be ready to go home. Once you are at home, the rest of your recovery and rehabilitation process will begin. It will be hard work – but the end result will be more mobility, less pain and greater freedom to do the activities you love.

SPECIAL ITEMS YOU MAY NEED BEFORE GOING HOME

To aid you in your recovery and care for your surgical wounds properly, you may need some special equipment for use at home. Talk with your doctor and nurses to find out if you will need these items and if there are any vendors or brands that they recommend:

- **TED hose** – These are the support stockings that you have probably been wearing in the hospital to prevent blood clots in your legs. Your doctor will likely recommend that you keep wearing these for the first few weeks after you leave the hospital. You will still have some swelling and will need to take care to prevent potentially dangerous clots. You can usually obtain TED hose at medical-supply stores.

- **Bandages and items for wound care** – Your nurse or doctor should give you instructions on how to care for your surgical wound and your stitches. Find out when you should change bandages and what type to use. Ask the nurse or doctor if you do not understand how to change your bandages. You may also need to have some type of antiseptic or antibiotic ointment for the wound. Ask your nurse or doctor if you need these items, how they should be used for bandage changes, and if they recommend any particular brands or types.

- **Crutches or a walker** – You may need help getting around your house at first after surgery. If necessary, your doctor will recommend a walker, crutches or a cane. Be sure you have the walking aid you need before leaving the hospital. Your doctor or the hospital nurse can help you arrange for these crucial supplies through a medical supply store or vendor. They can be delivered to the hospital or to your home.

- **Wheelchair** – You may need to have a wheelchair if you will need to go long distances from the car once you get home or on some other outing before you fully recover.

- **Other useful aids** – There are other helpful items you may wish to have on hand for use at home. You may wish to have a thermometer, and bedpan or bedside commode, as getting out of bed to go to the bathroom may be difficult at first. There are three-in-one commode seats that include a bedside commode, a raised toilet seat and a shower seat. A long-handled sponge, a bath or shower bench, and a handheld shower hose will be helpful for bathing because you will have to avoid getting your wound wet. A sock aid can help you put socks on before you are able to bend your leg all the way. A long-handled reacher can help you grasp items before you are able to move as you used to. An apron with pockets will allow you to carry items with you easily when you need hands for using crutches.

Leaving the Hospital

Even though you may have a walker or cane, chances are you won't be leaving the hospital on your own and hopping into your car after surgery. You will need to arrange to have a family member or trusted friend bring you home from the hospital. Be sure this person is strong enough to help you maneuver in and out of the car, or consider having two people help you.

You will usually be taken from the hospital to the car in a wheelchair. Take your time and maneuver slowly into the car. Open the door as wide as you can and adjust the seat so you have as much room as possible to get into the car without much bending of your leg. If you're apprehensive about getting into the car, ask if a nurse or physical therapist can be on hand to help you when you're discharged.

GOING HOME: WHAT TO EXPECT

Initially, going home will require some adjustments. But keep in mind that all of this is part of the process to greater mobility and less pain once you have recovered from the operation. You will need to take care to follow any precautions your doctor and therapist have given you for moving your joint. You also will need to carefully follow your exercise plan to make sure your joint heals properly and to regain your strength.

As you improve, you can gradually walk further or perform more activities around the house. Use your own judgment. Don't put yourself in a position where you might feel unsteady, frightened or stranded in one part of the house. Go slowly and do what you feel confident you can do.

It is important that you keep your new joint in mind whenever you move. While moving and regaining strength are important, you still need to take care of your fragile new joint. At first, don't move too quickly and think about your movements before you make them. You may have a tendency to want to move more quickly when you are comfortable at home rather than at the hospital.

You will also need to take care of your surgical wound. This will involve keeping it clean and dry to prevent infection and changing the bandages as needed. If your wound looks red or drains fluid, be sure to notify your doctor. You will also need to take your temperature periodically because a high temperature may be a sign of infection. Call your doctor if your temperature is higher than 101 degrees Fahrenheit.

You will have to watch for other signs of possible complications so you can notify your doctor. Keep an eye out for symptoms such as:

- Swelling that doesn't go away when you elevate the limb
- Pain behind your knee or in your calf
- Warmth and redness
- Chest pain
- Shortness of breath
- Coughing up blood
- Severe pain in your joint

Until you have your stitches removed, you may have to take sponge baths rather than showers or regular baths. Stitches or staples are usually removed two to three weeks after the operation.

TAKING MEDICATIONS PROPERLY

After surgery you will most likely have some medications to take, at least for the initial stage of your recovery. At first, this may include blood thinners, such as warfarin, to prevent blood clots from forming. You will also have some pain medication, some antibiotics to prevent infection, and perhaps sleep medication if you're having trouble sleeping.

Make sure that you understand all of your doctor's instructions for taking the medication – and follow them. Take your medications only as directed. If you have a question about one of the drugs you're taking, contact your doctor or pharmacist. Be sure that you know whether the drug is something you have to take until you have finished the course of pills you have been given (such as with an antibiotic), or if you can take the medication only as needed, which may be the case with pain medications. If you are not sure, ask your doctor.

To prevent possible infection once you have a joint implant, you may also need to take antibiotics before you have dental work done. Find out if your doctor recommends this preventive treatment, and be sure to notify your dentist before you have even routine procedures such as a cleaning.

LOOKING AHEAD

In this chapter we've reviewed what will take place during the surgical procedure itself. We've gone through the step, from checking in at the hospital, to the pre-operative procedures and surgery, to the post-surgical recovery. We've gone over the instruments the surgeon will use and the steps of the procedure. And we've taken you through the initial recovery from anesthesia and how you can expect to feel immediately after surgery.

Next, we'll take you through the longer-term recovery and what you can expect to face once you reach home. We'll examine some tips for making your recovery a smooth one and look at some of the challenges you'll face during this next stage of the surgery process and how to get through them.

chapter 10:

What Happens
During Recovery

After your operation, focusing on your recovery and everything that entails will be your job for the next several weeks. All the work you went through to prepare for surgery and get yourself through the procedure itself isn't over once you're in recovery. This part of the process also takes work and a commitment on your part. In fact, a great deal of the overall success of your surgery depends on how well the recovery process goes.

Not only does surgical recovery put stress on your body, it also puts stress on your emotions and relationships as well. Make sure that you and your family and friends are aware of the emotional challenges you'll face. (See page 94.) But know that you can get through the difficult parts of recovery. It may be tough for you at times, but if you're aware those challenges are coming, you can get yourself ready to take them on and more successfully push through them.

The Challenges of Recovery

While this part of the process involves a number of challenges, you will find the results well worth it in the end. Here we'll look at what your recovery includes, especially once you leave the hospital.

PHYSICAL THERAPY

A large part of the success of your operation will depend on your commitment to physical therapy during your recovery. This is the component of recovery that will allow you to make the most of your new joint by rebuilding your strength and learning to work with your new hip or knee.

Physical therapy focuses on helping people to improve their physical functioning and move more easily. As we learned on page 35, physical therapists are health professionals with specialized training in using physical methods, such as massage and exercise, to treat disease and help patients recover from surgery. These therapists typically have a master's degree in physical therapy.

After surgery, a physical therapist will provide you with specific instructions and exercises to follow to help you regain your strength, heal after surgery and regain mobility in your surgically repaired joint. Immediately after the operation, your joint and muscles will have some healing to do. You probably won't be able to move it very easily at first. Physical therapy will gradually help you to move it more easily, through exercises that rebuild the strength of the muscles and that take the joint through its range of motion.

The supervision and instructions from the physical therapist will help you to move your joint and exercise in the right way to avoid injuring yourself during the healing process. Physical therapy can also help you with methods to control pain, such as heat and cold treatments. (See more about heat and cold treatments on page 57.) Your physical therapist can also assist you in choosing devises to help you through recovery, such as a cane or walker and items to make bathing and dressing easier.

Like anything that can be time consuming and challenging, physical therapy after surgery requires your commitment and motivation. You may experience fatigue, some pain and even frustration, but you will have to remain focused on regaining the use of your joint.

You will likely have your first physical therapy appointment set up before you leave the hospital or very soon afterward. You may have sessions at home or at a rehabilitation center twice per week for several weeks. These sessions will include prescribed exercises that are specifically designed to help you regain the use of your joint. They will also help you rebuild muscle strength in your legs that can be affected by surgery.

You will need to perform these exercises diligently on your own as well. The physical therapy sessions will show you the correct way to do the exercises so you get the most benefit and don't harm yourself. In addition, your therapist can monitor your progress. You should also work on practical activities, such as walking, getting up from a chair, climbing stairs and other activities. You will learn to walk longer distances and gradually reduce your need for crutches or walking aids as you become stronger.

To help keep you motivated, try some ways that you can see the progress you have made. You may want to keep a journal of your recovery process. Make notes of what you are able to do at each therapy appointment. Take note of the new activities you can do each time, or how much further you can walk or move your joint. Your physical therapist can help point out some of the milestones. Keeping track in this way can give you a sense of accomplishment and allow you to see how far you've come. That can give you a boost to keep you going when the exercises seem tough.

PROTECTING YOUR JOINTS DURING RECOVERY

In most cases patients can get back to their usual activities within three to six weeks after surgery. During your recovery, and in some instances for the rest of your life, you will need to take certain precautions to protect your new joint.

For example, the hip joint can usually bend at angles greater than 90 degrees. But after hip replacement, your movement at first will be limited and you should not bend it at angles greater than 90 degrees. With new knees and new hips, your doctor may also limit the amount of weight you can put on them as well as the intensity of physical activities that you do. There are new types of knee replacement components that can bend up to 155 degrees. Ask your surgeon if you are eligible to receive this type of component.

At the same time you may need to adjust how you do certain activities or get some help with some of them until you fully recover. Following are some tips for handling daily activities after joint surgery.

DRESSING

To reduce some of the effort of getting dressed, you may want to plan ahead by picking out some loose fitting, easy-to-wear clothes that you have. Or you may want to pick up some elastic-waist pants or other pull-on clothing to wear during the first week or two after surgery.

You won't be able to bend your leg completely right after hip or knee surgery, so consider wearing slip-on shoes at first so you won't have to worry about tying laces. Long-handled shoehorns and sock aids are also helpful until you have more mobility in your leg. You also may need the assistance of your spouse, family member or close friend when getting dressed during the first few days after the operation.

BATHING/SHOWERING

Before your stitches are removed, you will need to make sure your incision stays dry. This can make bathing challenging. Try a bath seat and a shower hose to take a sponge-type bath. A long-handled sponge can help you clean areas that are hard to reach until you can move more easily.

Once your stitches are removed and you can shower, make sure you have grab bars to stead you or consider using a shower seat so you can prevent falls until you are steadier on your feet.

EATING AND DRINKING

To aid the healing process and the building of muscle strength, it is important for you to eat a healthful diet. You may lose your appetite for the first few days or weeks after the operation, but make sure you get the nutrition you need. When planning for your surgery, make sure you have someone available to help you prepare meals or that you have some easily heated meals on hand. Ask your doctor if he recommends an iron supplement to help with healing. Drink plenty of fluids as well.

MOVING AROUND THE HOUSE

You will be a bit unsteady for a while as you learn to use crutches and work to regain muscle strength. Be sure that you and the members of your household avoid leaving items on the floor that are easy to trip on. Remove throw rugs and electrical cords that could cause you to stumble. And think before you move.

A fall after surgery could be devastating. You could injure the surgical wounds that are healing or you could break a bone that surrounds an artificial joint. In that case, you could have to have the surgery repeated, which can be very difficult. It is best to be very careful to avoid falls after surgery.

Use your crutches or walker for stability as you walk and take advantage of handrails along staircases if you can. Place a pillow or cushion on low chairs so you don't have to bend as far to sit down.

GETTING OUT OF THE HOUSE

For a short time after surgery, you may not be able to drive a car. How long this lasts may depend on what type of surgery you have. You should ask your doctor about how long you should wait before trying to drive. Although people today are very dependent on their cars for getting where they need to go, driving requires that you have quick physical responses and enough strength and dexterity to operate the vehicle safely.

Until you can drive again, you will need a friend or family member to take you where you need to go. You may also consider taxicabs for emergencies, or explore community-based car services. Some community centers or charities operate driving services for people who need to get to medical appointments and other necessary trips.

When entering cars, make it easier on yourself by having the seat all the way back so you have plenty of room to maneuver. Carefully lower yourself to the seat, slide back and pivot your legs in front of you. Consider using a swivel-seat attachment (available through assistive device catalogs or retailers) to help you slide in and out of the car seat. Be sure to have your walker, cane or crutches with you to help you get around.

A Note on Assistive Devices

Throughout this section we have mentioned some assistive devices, daily living aids and adaptive equipment that may be helpful to you during your recovery from surgery. You can obtain these items from a number of resources.

First, ask your physical therapist, who can tell you which items will be most useful to you and can likely recommend a local store where you can find them. You can also check your phone book for local medical supply stores. There are also numerous catalogs that sell these items, allowing you to order over the phone or from their Web site and shipping the items directly to your home. Try searching for medical supply or adaptive equipment companies, or ask your physical therapist for the name of a reputable company. Your physical therapist is likely to have copies of the catalogs and may be able to loan or give you a copy.

Check your insurance plan to find out if it covers these daily living aids. In some cases, if you need your doctor or physical therapist's recommendation or prescription, your insurance may cover it. Find out what is covered before you purchase the items.

ASKING FOR HELP

While you are recovering, don't try to do everything yourself. Asking for help should not be considered a sign of weakness or a lack of self-reliance. Your friends and family know you are recovery, and they want to help you get well. Don't hesitate or be afraid to ask for their help when you need it. You will be aiding your recovery if you don't do too much too soon and avoid hurting yourself.

At the same time, keep in mind that you shouldn't be exceedingly demanding either. Of course your friends and family want to help, but try to make it easy for them and convenient when you can. If you need a ride somewhere and you don't need to go immediately, ask when they are going in that direction or try to combine trips you need to make. If you need a couple of favors, ask when it would be convenient, if the tasks can wait, rather than asking for several favors in succession. Sometimes your need can't wait, but try to plan ahead if you can.

Here are some additional tips on asking for help:
- Ask for specific help so the person knows what you need.
- Have a group of family and friends you can call on, instead of relying on just one or two people.
- Offer help to them in return with tasks you can do. Or promise to return the favor once you're fully recovered.

PREVENTING INFECTION

Taking steps to prevent infection after joint surgery is very important. Infections can enter your body in a number of ways, and even a minor one can be very dangerous when you have an artificial joint. Infections can occur in joint implants any time after surgery, so you will need to continue prevention efforts.

If an infection reaches your artificial joint through your bloodstream, you may require intense treatment and you may need to have an infected implant removed and replaced in another operation. Though this type of deep infection is rare, you should still take precautions. If you

Signs of an Infection

Signs of Infection Include:

- Fever
- Redness or swelling of a wound
- Drainage from a wound
- Increased pain in a joint during activity and rest

You Can Prevent Infection by:

- Keeping wounds clean. Your doctor or a nurse will give you specific instructions on how to keep your surgical wound clean after surgery and on how and when to change bandages or dressings. You should avoid soaking in a tub or getting the wound wet until it has healed.

- Taking antibiotics before dental procedures and other medical procedures such as gynecological exams and minor surgical procedures

- Talking with your physician if you suspect or see signs of an infection so it can be treated promptly

believe you have an infection, notify your doctor right away. See the box on page 178 for some common signs of an infection and what you should do if you notice these signs.

Once you have an artificial joint, be sure to notify your dentist and other doctors that you have a joint implant before you have any procedures done, including minor ones like teeth cleaning. Even during a routine dental examination, you might run the risk of an infection. Even a small infection can become a major problem if you have an artificial joint, but your health-care professionals know what precautions to take. It's up to you to keep them informed about your new joint!

LOOKING AHEAD

In this chapter, we've learned what you can expect to experience during your recovery from surgery. We've looked at how physical therapy will help you to regain mobility and use of your joint during your recovery as well as the care you'll need to take with your surgical wound and surgically repaired joint. We've also learned important ways you can prevent infection after surgery.

Next, we'll explore your long-term recovery from surgery and how you can get your life back in order. We'll also learn about how soon you can expect to resume your usual activities.

chapter 11:

Getting Your
Life Back in Order

Joint surgery and recovery probably sounds like a long process – and it is a long process with lots of things to think about, take care of and do. You may wonder how long it will be after your surgery before you are back to your old self. How long will it take for you to recover and rehabilitate your joint to the point where you are free to do the things you enjoy, or handle daily activities like driving, shopping or cooking on your own without help.

In this chapter we will examine the process of getting back into normal activities, and explore how soon you can resume your usual tasks. You can rest assured that despite the recovery and rehabilitation necessary after joint surgery, this time will be here before you know it!

When Can You
Resume Normal Activities?

Resuming your normal activities will probably be a gradual process. As you rebuild muscle strength and improve flexibility in your new joint, you will feel ready to do more things. If you have a concern about a specific activity and when it is safe for you to resume, talk with your doctor or physical therapist.

Your doctor and physical therapist can assess the progress you have made with your rehabilitation. These professionals can tell you about any precautions or dangers. Depending on the type of surgery you've had, you may be able to being more strenuous activities, such as swimming or bicycling, by about six weeks after surgery. Some procedures require longer recovery time.

DRIVING

Because driving requires you to bear weight on your leg, you will have to regain your strength enough to accomplish that goal first. Driving also requires you to have upper-body mobility, and hand and finger dexterity (to steer, operate the controls, turn around to back up), so if you have had surgery that affects your arms, hands, fingers or shoulders, it may be some time before you rehabilitate your mobility and dexterity in those areas.

Many people will regain strength in their legs by six to eight weeks after a knee or hip operation. You must also be finished using any narcotic pain medications, which should not be taken if you are driving. Your ability to drive also depends on which joint you have had replaced. If you use your right leg to drive and you have had surgery on the left leg, you may be able to drive a little sooner than if you had had surgery on the right leg. Keep in mind that you will still need to be careful of your hip or knee when getting in and out of the car.

SELF-CARE AND GROOMING

As mentioned earlier, you should avoid taking baths or showers until your stitches or staples are removed. You will have your stitches or staples removed about two to three weeks after the operation.

To avoid falls in the bath or shower, make sure that you can be steady on your feet and that you have a nonslip surface in the tub or shower, such as a suction-cup mat or special nonslip stickers you can place on the bottom of the shower. (These are good things to have in your tub or shower anyway!) You can find these items at home supply or bath stores. If you are uncertain, use a bath or shower seat or have a family member assist you in getting in and out of the shower.

Approximately four to six weeks after surgery, your surgeon will take X-rays to evaluate your progress. This will help determine which activities you can safely do. Your doctor will tell you whether you've healed enough to safely resume certain activities.

OTHER ACTIVITIES

Most people can resume many other activities, such as golfing, dancing, bicycling and swimming, about six to eight weeks after the typical surgery. You'll need to avoid high impact activities or those that put stress on your knee or hip, such as tennis, heavy lifting, contact sports, skiing and jogging.

Certain types of implants can affect this timing as well. With uncemented hip implants, you should avoid putting weight on the leg for six weeks and then gradually bear weight on the leg a little at a time while still using a walking aid.

SEX

Most people can safely resume sexual activity about four to six weeks after surgery. Talk to your doctor about any precautions you should take with your artificial joint, such as body positions that could be painful or harmful.

Although you can safely kneel once the tissues in your knee have healed, you may still prefer positions that avoid direct pressure on your knees. For hip replacements, avoid positions that cause you to sit with your knees higher than your hips, that cause your knees to touch, or that cause your leg and foot to roll inward.

The Arthritis Foundation offers a free publication, *A Guide to Intimacy With Arthritis,* that explores ways to engage in sex without harming your joints, or sexual positions that accommodate people with joint problems or mobility problems. This publication is available by calling 800/283-7800 or online at www.arthritis.org. If you have specific questions or concerns, ask your doctor or physical therapist.

WORK

The type of work you do will affect how soon you can return to work. If you have a desk job that has very few physical demands, you may be able to return to work as early as six weeks after your operation. You may need to make sure you can move around periodically, though, so your joint does not become too stiff.

If your job calls for long periods of standing, walking or lifting, you may need to wait 12 weeks before returning to ensure that your joint is properly healed to withstand the strain. You may be able to return earlier than that if you can scale back these activities significantly at first.

Talk to your surgeon or physical therapist about the types of tasks your job requires and consider seeing an occupational therapist as well. Occupational therapists focus on helping you achieve the best possible function and on modifying daily activities. They may be able to recommend certain ways to modify tasks or adaptive equipment that could allow you to do your job while protecting your new joint.

Exercise

Exercise is an important part not only of your recovery, but also of keeping your new joint and your other joints in the best possible shape. During your recovery, exercise will be necessary for regaining your mobility. You can continue the routine you establish during this time into your post-recovery life. If you have chosen a certain time of day to perform your physical therapy exercises or gradually push your walking distance a little further, continue to make that your exercise time. Just as you make time for it in your recovery, make time for it in the rest of your life.

After joint surgery, some types of exercise are more suitable for you than others. Injury to your joint is a risk after surgery. The implant could become dislocated, possibly requiring additional surgery to correct it. Or you could fall and possibly break the bone around the implant, which could also lead to revision surgery. Before you begin an activity or exercise program, talk to your doctor or surgeon about what is appropriate.

In general, activities that are gentle and that don't put too much strain or impact on your joint are more suitable than high-impact ones. Walking, golfing, swimming, biking and dancing are all appropriate activities after hip or knee replacement. If you have had shoulder replacement, check with your doctor to find out if playing golf is OK.

Most doctors recommend avoiding jogging, skiing, playing tennis and playing basketball.

Other gentle sports such as yoga and tai chi are also good options, with proper supervision. If you are interested in taking an exercise class, you may wish to talk to the exercise instructor to let him or her know you have had joint surgery. Ask the instructor if this type of exercise is acceptable for your needs. Don't risk an injury later if you can get some information ahead of time.

WATER EXERCISE

Another appropriate type of gentle exercise is water exercise, such as the Arthritis Foundation's Aquatics Program (AFAP). This popular course is given at pools around the country, as well as at YMCAs, where it is known as AFYAP (Arthritis Foundation YMCA Aquatics Program). Your local Arthritis Foundation chapter can guide you to the nearest certified aquatics course. Find your local office by calling 800/283-7800 or by logging on to www.arthritis.org.

AFAP is designed to increase your range of motion and dexterity, as well as building strength and cardiovascular fitness. This soothing form of exercise uses resistance from the water to achieve a good workout. At the same time, the water provides support by holding your body afloat. This type of exercise is highly recommended for people with arthritis as well as joint replacements because it provides the right amount of activity without stressing and straining joints. The Arthritis Foundation also sells a home video version of the program (if you have your own pool or access to one in your neighborhood) called PEP (Pool Exercise Program). Call 800/207-8633 to order, or log on to www.arthritis.org.

SAMPLE EXERCISES

These exercises are designed to strengthen the muscles around your joints. Several of these moves may be similar to those recommended as pre-surgery exercises. Before you begin, talk to your doctor and physical therapist about which specific exercises are right for you.

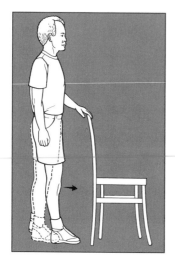

1. Hip flexion

Stand with your feet slightly apart and your hands resting on the back of a chair. Move the leg that had surgery forward while keeping your knee straight. Then move it back to the starting position. You can add resistance by placing an elastic exercise band around your ankles. Repeat the exercise with your other leg.

2. Side leg lift

Stand next to a chair with your hand resting on the back for support. Using your leg that had surgery, move it out to the side. Then return your leg to the starting position. You can add resistance here with an elastic exercise band as well. Repeat the exercise with your other leg.

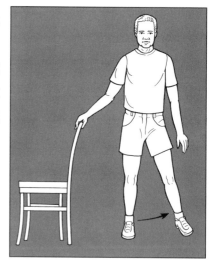

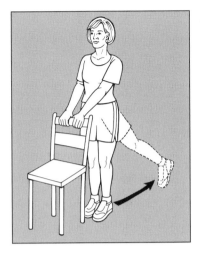

3. Back kick

Stand with your hands resting on the back of a chair. Move the leg that had surgery backward behind you, then return it to the starting position. An elastic exercise band can add resistance to this exercise too. Repeat the exercise with your other leg.

4. Leg raises

Lie on your back and bend one knee. Lift your straight leg slowly a few inches and hold for 5 seconds. Then lower your leg. Repeat a few times, then switch legs.

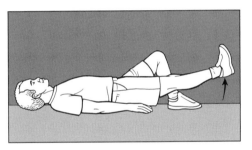

KEEPING WEIGHT OFF

Just as it was important to be in good shape for surgery, it is also important to continue after you have your new joint. Extra pounds add more strain to joints, so keeping excess weight off after surgery is important for keeping your new joint functioning well.

In addition to exercising regularly, you should continue to follow the healthy eating plan that you may have started in order to lose weight for surgery. (Review the information in Chapter 7.) If you have already been eating a healthful diet for some time, keep it up. All of your joints will feel better for it.

There are no foods proven to cause or worsen joint inflammation or pain, despite some of the claims made in books, health news and other sources. The most important thing you can do to maintain healthy joints is to eat a balanced, healthy diet and keep your weight under control. Extra pounds will stress your joints – not the content of any food.

LOOKING AHEAD

In this chapter, we've examined the long-term recovery process, in particular how you can recover your life after your joint has begun healing. We've looked at how soon you'll be able to resume normal activities, such as driving, working, exercising and having sex. We've also seen ways that you can keep your joints healthy, such as through exercise and keeping off excess weight. In the next chapter, we'll look at what you can expect in the months and years after your surgery and recovery are complete.

chapter 12:

What To Expect
in the Long Term

Now that you have made it through the operation and the recovery, you have a new joint to enjoy with less pain and improved function. While your surgically repaired joint should feel much better and allow you to move more easily, keep in mind that you will not feel as if you never had arthritis or an injury to your joint.

Joint surgery does not "cure" joint problems or arthritis. You may not necessarily be able to do any activity that you dream about without some limitations. But you can expect to feel a good deal of improvement after your recovery and you should be able to resume some activities that you had difficulty doing before.

In this chapter, we'll look at what you can expect from your surgically repaired joint in more detail. How can you expect that joint to hold up in the long run? We will look into that question and several other long-term concerns now.

Long-Term Use of Your Surgically Repaired Joint

Joint surgery is designed to help you experience less pain and improve your ability to move. For most people, joint surgery accomplishes those very goals.

For example, about 90 percent of people who have knee replacement surgery have a major reduction in pain and a much greater ability to perform daily activities. For others, arthroscopic surgery provides great relief and allows them to get back to their lives quickly. You may find that after surgery you can walk longer distances without pain, you may be able to play a light game of tennis or golf again, or you may have an easier time getting dressed or doing household tasks without help from others. You may find that after recovery from knee surgery, you no longer have pain in your knee while going up and down stairs.

Keep in mind that despite the highly sophisticated surgical procedures, much of the success of surgery depends on you. Your commitment to regaining movement and performing your physical therapy exercises during the first few weeks of recovery can have tremendous influence on your overall outcome. Take advantage of your chance to make the most of your recovery through the aspects you can control.

You will also need to remember to take care of your new or repaired joint. You will have to protect it from falls and exercise safely to keep it healthy. You also should avoid very high impact or overly stressful activities that could damage your newly repaired joint. By following these precautions, you can enjoy the benefits of joint surgery.

WHAT IS THE CHANCE OF FAILURE?

For the most part, people who are deemed appropriate candidates for joint surgery generally have good outcomes from it. In fact, joint replacement surgery is considered to be a very successful type of surgery.

Despite the positive record of success with these operations, problems can arise for some patients. There are always risks associated with surgery. Here are some of the problems to watch out for over the long term. If you feel you are experiencing one of these, or something doesn't feel right about your implant, let your doctor or surgeon know so they can evaluate what is happening right away.

For some people, arthroscopy may have to be performed again. Because this method can be used to look inside a joint to assess what is happening, if you experience more pain down the road, your doctor may recommend arthroscopy again to get a better view of what is happening in the joint. Or in some cases, perhaps not all of a damaged piece of cartilage is removed so the operation may have to be repeated to trim an additional portion of cartilage that may be causing pain.

For people with RA who have a synovectomy surgery to remove a diseased joint lining, the surgery does not cure the underlying process of rheumatoid arthritis. Rheumatoid arthritis is a chronic disease for which there currently is no cure (although there are many new, highly effective treatments). After surgery, the synovium can grow back and may still be diseased, so it may have to be removed again at a future date.

Loosening

Most joint replacements are designed to last for 15 to 20 years, and new technology is being developed all the time to help them last even longer. But sometimes the components of joint implants can loosen over time, in some cases causing pain. This problem can occur if the implant isn't secured well enough with bone cement or, in a cement-less implant, if surrounding bone doesn't grow well enough to hold the prosthesis in place properly. If the problem is severe enough, joint replacement surgery may have to be redone.

Bone Loss

Sometimes as an implant wears over time, loose particles of material can be released into your body. These particles can cause reactions in your body that in some cases can cause bone loss called **osteolysis**. If the problem is extensive enough, more surgery may be required to replace the implant and prevent further bone loss.

For some people, less invasive types of surgery may be a way of putting off total joint replacement. Many times this can buy you some time by relieving pain for a significant period of time. But the surgical procedures do not change how arthritis operates in your body. Your joint may still deteriorate further even after you have surgery if you have arthritis.

A less invasive type of surgery may provide relief and improvement for a while, but some people may eventually need to have joint replacement surgery anyway. In addition, arthroscopy frequently is used as a diagnostic procedure as well as a treatment procedure. You may need an additional arthroscopic procedure down the road if your doctor needs to see the inside of your joint or treat a portion of the cartilage.

WHAT IS REPEAT SURGERY LIKE?

In general terms, the procedure for revision surgery is very much like that of the original surgery. However, several factors can make revision surgery more challenging. The operation can be more complex with a greater risk of complications, such as infection or dislocation, because the patient is usually older than during the original surgery and because the second surgery is more involved. This may mean additional types of preparation beforehand, such as a more lengthy medical examination. Also, more blood will likely be needed because the procedure is longer.

The general procedure of implanting the new joint is relatively the same, but there are some differences in the overall procedure. First, the old implant has to be removed, which can be tricky and take time. Also, damaged bone may have to be repaired before the new implant can be placed. The implanting of the new joint, though, follows the same steps as the original procedure.

In addition, the patient may have lost bone or had other significant damage to the joint that may require additional repair or a larger implant to take the place of lost tissue or bone. Removing the first implant can also be difficult. All of these issues mean that revision surgery usually requires a longer operation and a longer recovery period. For example, the overall recovery from revision surgery may take up to a year. The difficulties also may mean that the outcome of revision surgery is not as good as that of the original operation. The new replacement joint may not work as well.

MAKING YOUR SURGERY A SUCCESS

There are steps you can take to increase the changes that your surgery is successful. One is by preparing yourself well ahead of time, as this book has taught you to do. Another is by carefully following your rehabilitation plan and dedicating yourself to it. That will help make sure that your joint heals properly and that the muscles around it become strong to support the joint well.

Finally, you can take precautions and take care of your new or repaired joint. Take care to avoid activities that can jeopardize or harm your joint, such as high impact or risky sports, or even unsafe everyday movements that your surgeon has advised you against.

For example, sports that require you to put the full weight of your body on one leg, such as jogging, are considered high impact and should be avoided. (See the list of sports or physical activities that may cause joint damage on page 30.) When you've had surgery on a knee or hip, avoid twisting your knee or hip too much and avoid very heavy lifting, which puts pressure on the large joints of your legs.

Take measures to prevent falls as well. A severe fall could cause you to loosen the implant or to fracture a bone around the implant. If the bone breaks above the implant, the implant often has to be replaced, particularly with a cemented implant. You can prevent falls by taking care to think before you move and to move more carefully in general.

Avoid quick turns and pivots or sudden changes in direction when possible. Take advantage of handrails, or use a cane if you are unsteady on your feet. Wear sensible shoes that don't snag or slip. At home, remove electrical cords from pathways that could cause tripping, and remove throw rugs or secure them to the floor. Keep pathways clear of objects and make your home well lit at night (consider using nightlights to light a pathway to the bathroom at night).

LOOKING AHEAD

In this chapter, we've looked at the long-term expectations after joint surgery, as well as some of the complications that could come up. We've also looked at how important it is to live a healthy lifestyle and avoid activities and habits that could negatively affect your joint surgery outcome. The advice covered in this chapter should help you to work toward long-term success of your joint surgery. Next, we'll look at how a new or repaired joint fits into your overall lifestyle, as well as resources that can help you.

chapter 13:

In Conclusion:
Life After Surgery

This book should provide you with a good foundation and guide as you deal with the prospect of joint surgery. Undergoing surgery is a major challenge, but you can make it through and come out with less pain and the ability to enjoy activity for the long term.

Getting on With Your Life

A few months after surgery (maybe less time with less invasive procedures), you should be feeling like you are on your way back to normal. You will have completed your rehabilitation plan and will have returned to work and resumed many of your usual activities. That's quite an achievement, and one that you should be proud to have accomplished.

Now that you have made it through surgery and recovery, you can get back to living your life and feel better doing the things you love to do.

LIMITATIONS YOU MAY EXPERIENCE

While you are the outcome of your operation should improve how you feel, you may not feel completely brand new. And although your new or repaired joint should function much better, you may still have some limitations. If you have had knee surgery, you may feel some discomfort with certain movements such as kneeling or lots of bending. Or you might feel a slight difference when you walk compared with how your leg felt before the implant.

In some cases joint implants can trigger airport or building security systems, so be sure to notify personnel that you have a joint replacement. It may be a good idea to ask your doctor to write you a note explaining that you have a joint implant in case an airport security device senses it. After the events of September 11, 2001, airport security measures have increased, and airport security agents may be more vigilant than ever about security risks. So be prepared to explain your joint implant and cooperate with any security measures.

ACHIEVING YOUR GOALS

Perhaps your only reason for having joint surgery was pain relief. But perhaps you also wanted to get back to an activity you had to give up because of pain. Or maybe there was some new activity you wanted to try, but couldn't because of arthritis. Even if your goals are just to be able to do everyday tasks like walking to the mailbox more easily, you can work toward them now.

Make your plans and work out the steps you will need to take to get there. Then make your progress through those steps until you reach your goal. Breaking it down into a series of steps makes the task seem less daunting and gives you a progressive set of achievements to keep you motivated. Tell your family and friends about your goals so they can encourage you and cheer with you when you reach them.

As you move forward in the long run of your recovery from surgery, keep in mind these important guidelines for joint health and overall health:

- **Exercise** – This all-important healthy habit played a major role in your preparation and recovery, and now it plays a major role in your continuing joint health. Make a commitment to regular exercise and stick with it. If you start to get bored or lack motivation, try something new or find a way to challenge yourself with new goals. There are many different ways to exercise. You need to try various activities to find what works for you and your schedule.

  A great way to stay fit after surgery without damaging your joints is walking. The Arthritis Foundation publishes a great guide to developing an effective, self-directed walk-for-fitness program called *Walk With Ease: Your Guide to Walking for Better Health, Improved Fitness and Less Pain*. While the book is designed to accommodate people with arthritis, it's an easy program that will increase anybody's fitness and overall health. Call 800/207-8633 to order, or order online at www.arthritis.org. All proceeds benefit the programs of the Arthritis Foundation. See the Resources for Good Living section at the end of this book for more information on Arthritis Foundation healthy products.

- **Diet**. Keeping extra pounds off is a great way to protect your joints from excess stress. Make your operation a success by staying fit through a healthful, balanced diet. Excess weight is a major con-tributing factor to osteoarthritis, particularly of the hips and knees, because the weight puts undue stress on these already hard-work-ing joints. A diet that is low in fat and cholesterol and high in fiber and nutrients will contribute to better overall health.

The Arthritis Foundation has a new book to help you make changes in diet and fitness and stick to them: *Change Your Life: Simple Strategies To Lose Weight, Get Fit and Improve Your Outlook.* The book contains guidelines and recipes, simple exercise techniques and stress-control tips to help you keep body and mind in balance. To order, call 800/207-8633 or order online at www.arthritis.org.

For more information on creating a healthful diet, explore the American Dietetic Assocation's Web site at www.eatright.org.

- **Not Smoking**. Along with your other commitments to health like diet and exercise, avoid smoking too. Smoking can contribute to a variety of serious health problems and will keep you from having a healthy lifestyle. It's also more difficult to recover from injuries or surgery when you smoke. There are many new, effective treatments available to help you quit smoking if you currently smoke. For more information on the dangers of smoking and tips for quitting, contact your doctor or the American Lung Association, www.lungusa.org.

- **Moderate Drinking**. Another step to overall good health is drinking alcohol only in moderation. Excess alcohol consumption can contribute to many health problems and can add excess, nutrition-empty calories to your diet. Drinking in moderation is preferable; ask your doctor to recommend specific amounts to keep within "moderate" bounds.

- **Stress Reduction**. Relaxing and managing stress in positive ways are important to your overall well-being. Find constructive ways to manage stress and use relaxation techniques when you feel overwhelmed. If you find that your stress is out of control – particularly if you are experiencing frequent anxiety, panic attacks, sleeplessness, headaches or are indulging in stress-related binge eating or smoking – it might be helpful to see a mental-health professional. Ask your physician to make a recommendation and see if your insurance policy covers visits to a mental-health professional or counseling service. Stress does not have to take over your life. By learning ways to release and control stress, you will create a healthier overall lifestyle with more activity.

In conclusion, we hope that *All You Need To Know About Joint Surgery* has helped you become more informed about these increasingly common surgical procedures. Preparation and knowledge are two of the most important tools you can have when you are having an operation of any kind, particularly joint surgery. If you do go forward with plans for joint surgery, we wish you success. Please consider the Arthritis Foundation as a resource of information and support during your surgery and in years to come.

GLOSSARY

A

Acetabulum – The socket of the hipbone, shaped like a cup, where the ball-shaped end of the femur (thighbone) fits.

Acetaminophen – Common analgesic or pain-fighting medicine. The most common brand name is *Tylenol*.

Acupressure – Eastern medicine technique in which pressure is applied to specific sites along energy pathways called meridians.

Acupuncture – Eastern medicine technique in which needles are used to puncture the body at specific sites along energy pathways called meridians.

Acute illness – Disease that can be severe but is of short duration, unlike chronic illness.

Acute pain – See *pain*.

Aerobic – An activity designed to increase oxygen consumption by the body, such as aerobic exercise or aerobic breathing.

Alternative therapy – Any practice or substance outside the realm of conventional medicine.

American College of Rheumatology (ACR) – An organization that provides a professional, educational, and research forum for rheumatologists across the country. Among its functions is helping determine what symptoms and signs define the various types of rheumatic disease diagnoses and what the appropriate treatments are for those diagnoses.

Analgesic – Drugs used to help relieve pain.

Anesthesia – Chemicals that induce a partial or complete loss of sensation. Used to perform surgery and other medical procedures.

Anesthesiologist – A physician specializing in the administration of anesthesia.

Antibiotics – Drugs used to inhibit the growth of various bacteria and other microorganisms that cause infectious diseases.

Antioxidants – Substances present in certain foods that protect the body from damage caused by harmful *free radicals*, molecules that are the by-products of cell metabolism. Foods rich in antioxidants help to slow the deterioration caused by these free radicals. See *free radicals.*

Arthritis – A disease generally involving pain or inflammation of a joint from any cause, such as infection, trauma or inflammation.

Arthrodesis – A surgical procedure involving the fusing of two bones.

Arthroplasty – A surgical procedure to replace a joint with an artificial one.

Arthroscopy – A type of surgery using an instrument, called an *arthroscope,* consisting of a thin tube with a light at one end, inserted into the body through a small incision, and connected to a closed-circuit television.

Aspiration – The removal of a substance by suction; a technique used to remove fluid from an inflamed joint, both to relieve pressure and to examine the fluid.

ASU – A mixture of avocado and soybean oils, taken as a dietary supplement and purported to ease osteoarthritis pain.

Autoimmune disease – A disease, such as rheumatoid arthritis, that

GLOSSARY

involves a malfunction of the body's immune system.

Autologous blood transfusion – A process where a surgery patient donates his or her own blood for use in transfusion during the operation.

B

Ball-and-socket joints – Joints such as the hips or shoulders that consist of a bone with a ball-shaped ending that fits into a round socket. This construction lets the bones to twist and turn in many directions while staying in place.

Biologic response modifiers – A new class of arthritis drugs that target specific chemicals in the immune system known as cytokines, which play a role in inflammation and damage, but leave other parts of the immune system intact.

Body mechanics – The structures and methods with which your body moves and performs physical tasks.

Bone spur – Bony outgrowths (also called osteophytes) that occur when bones in a joint thicken and change due to the cartilage break-down common in arthritis.

Boron – A trace mineral that helps the body use nutrients like calcium and magnesium. Taken as a supplement, it is purported to ease osteoarthritis symptoms.

Boswellia – Also known as frankincense, derived from an Asian tree. Combined with other herbs, it is purported to ease osteoarthritis symptoms.

Bunion – Inflammation, enlargement and malalignment of the joint of the great toe.

Bursa – A small sac located between a tendon and a bone. The bursae (plural for bursa) reduce friction and provide lubrication. See also *bursitis*.

Bursitis – Inflammation of a bursa (see *bursa* above), which can occur when the joint has been overused or when the joint has become deformed by arthritis. Bursitis makes it painful to move or put pressure on the affected joint.

C

Capsaicin – A chemical contained in some hot peppers. Capsaicin gives these peppers their "burn" and has painkilling properties. It is available in nonprescription creams that can be rubbed on the skin over a joint to relieve pain.

Cartilage – A firm, smooth, rubbery substance that provides a gliding surface for joint motion, and prevents bone-on-bone contact.

Catheter – A slender, hollow tube inserted into a body cavity or passage in order to drain fluid, examine the body, or infuse drugs; commonly used in surgery to help drain urine from the bladder.

Cemented/cementless implant – Term that refers to two different techniques for holding a joint replacement component in place during total joint replacement surgery; "cemented" refers to the use of an adhesive, and "cementless" refers to a technique where bone grows around the replacement to hold it in place.

Chiropractic – Practice of healing based on spinal manipulation and the belief that illness stems from misalignment of the spinal cord.

Chiropractor – Also known as a doctor of chiropractic, a health professional certified in chiropractic; these professionals are not licensed to perform surgery or prescribe drugs.

Chondroitin sulfate – Dietary supplement derived from cattle trachea, purported to help stop joint degeneration, improve function and ease pain; part of a naturally occurring protein in human cartilage that gives cartilage elasticity.

Chronic illness – Disease that is of a long duration, such as rheumatoid arthritis.

GLOSSARY

Chronic pain – Pain that is constant or persists over a long period of time, perhaps throughout life. See *pain*.

Collagen – A protein that is the primary component of cartilage (see *cartilage*).

Complementary therapy – Any practice or substance used in conjunction with traditional treatment; also known as *alternative therapy*.

Continuous passive motion machine – An apparatus used in the hospital just after surgery to help the patient move and exercise the limb that has been operated on.

Corticosteroids: See *glucocorticoids*.

Cortisone – A hormone produced by the cortex of the adrenal gland. Cortisone has potent anti-inflammatory effects but can also have side effects. See also *glucocorticoids*.

Counterirritants – Topical analgesics that contain substances such as oil of wintergreen, camphor or eucalyptus oil, which stimulate nerve endings and distract the brain from joint pain.

COX-2 drugs – Also known as COX-2 inhibitors, drugs that inhibit inflammation with a reduced risk of gastrointestinal side effects of traditional NSAIDs. Includes celecoxib, rofecoxib and valdecoxib.

Deep-tissue massage – Massage technique in which a therapist uses fingers, thumbs and elbows to put strong pressure on deep muscles and tissue layers to relieve chronic tension.

Dietitian – Professional who advises people on diet matters, such as meal planning or weight loss.

Directed blood transfusion – Type of blood transfusion used in surgery in which the patient receives blood donated from another person, rather than his or her own blood.

Disease – Sickness; some physicians use this term only for conditions in which a structural or functional change in tissues or organs has been identified.

Disease-modifying antirheumatic drugs: Class of drugs used to modify the course of joint damage in rheumatoid arthritis, slowing or even stopping its progression.

Disorder – An ailment; an abnormal health condition.

E

Endorphins – Natural painkillers produced by the human nervous system that have qualities similar to opiate drugs. Endorphins are released during exercise and when we laugh.

Endurance exercises – Exercises such as swimming, walking and cycling that use the large muscles of the body and are dependent on increasing the amount of oxygen that reaches the muscles. These exercises strengthen muscles and increase and maintain physical fitness.

Epidural – A form of anesthesia where a small dose of an anesthetic drug is injected into the epidural space in the lower back, near the spinal column.

Ergonomics – The study of human capabilities and limitations in relation to the work system, machine or task, as well as the study of the physical, psychological and social environment of the worker; also known as "human engineering".

F

Facet joints – Joints such as those of the spine whose construction allows bones to twist, turn or rotate for a broad range of motion.

Fatigue – A general worn-down feeling of no energy. Fatigue can be caused by excessive physical, mental or emotional exertion, by lack of sleep, and by inflammation or disease.

GLOSSARY

Flare – A term used to describe times when a disease or condition is at its worst.

Flexibility exercises – Muscle stretches and other activities designed to maintain flexibility and to prevent stiffness or shortening of ligaments and tendons.

Food Labeling Act – Recent legal decree of the U.S. government mandating the type of information that must be given on food labels regarding nutritional content. This Act ensures that consumers will have easy-to-read fat, protein, fiber, carbohydrate and calorie content information, and more. See *USDA Food Guide Pyramid*.

Free radicals – Molecules that are the by-products of cell deterioration; believed to contribute to some damage or disease in the body.

G

Ginger – Root that, when taken in the form of tea or supplement cap-

sules, is purported to relieve pain and inflammation.

Glucocorticoids – A group of hormones including cortisol produced by the adrenal glands. They can also be synthetically produced (that is, made in a laboratory) and have powerful anti-inflammatory effects.

Glucosamine – An amino sugar that appears to play a role in cartilage formation and repair. Taken as a dietary supplement derived from crab, lobster and shrimp shells, it is purported to relieve pain.

Hinge joints – Joints such as knees or elbows that move back and forth like an opening and closing door's hinge.

Home health aide – Nurse or nursing aide hired to assist with care or recovery in one's home after surgery or during a serious illness.

Hormones – Concentrated chemical substances produced in the glands or organs that have specific – and usually multiple – regulatory effects to carry out in the body.

Hyaluronan – A substance, also called hyaluronic acid, in the synovial fluid of the joint, giving it viscosity and helping the joint absorb shock.

Hypertension – Another term for high blood pressure.

I

Illness – Poor health; sickness

Inflammation – A response to injury or infection that involves a sequence of biochemical reactions. Inflammation can be generalized, causing fatigue, fever, and pain or tenderness all over the body. It can also be localized, for example, in joints, where it causes swelling and pain.

Informed consent – Term referring to an official form or forms indicating that a surgery patient entering the hospital understands and accepts the treatment he or she is scheduled to receive.

Internist – A physician who specializes in internal medicine; sometimes called a primary-care physician.

Isometric exercises – Exercises that build the muscles around joints by tightening the muscles without moving the joints.

Isotonic exercises – Exercises that strengthen muscles by moving the joints.

J

Joint – The place or part where one bone connects to another.

Joint aspiration – Also known as arthrocentesis, a laboratory test where fluid is drained from the joint and examined for crystals or joint deterioration.

GLOSSARY

Joint capsule – Area where components of the joint come together

Joint fluid therapy – Injecting hyaluronic acid into a joint.

Joint malalignment – When joints are not aligned properly, due to joint damage

Joint replacement surgery – Also known as arthroplasty, a surgical procedure involving the reconstruction or replacement (with a man-made component) of a joint

Ligament – Flexible band of fibrous tissue that connects bones to one another.

Massage – A technique of applying pressure, friction or vibration to the muscles, by hand or using a massage appliance, to stimulate circu-

lation and produce relaxation and pain relief.

Meridians – Energy pathways used in Eastern medicine, but that have no Western medicine counterparts.

Muscle – Tissue that moves organs or parts of the body.

Myalgia – Pain of the muscles.

Myofascial release – A massage technique in which the therapist applies slow, steady pressure to relieve tension in the fascia, or the thin tissue around the muscles.

Neuromuscular massage – A massage technique in which the therapist uses fingers and thumbs to massage points in the body (trigger points) which may trigger pain in other areas of the body.

NSAID (nonsteroidal anti-inflammatory drug) – A type of drug that does not contain steroids but is used to relieve pain and reduce inflammation.

Nurse – A person who has received education and training in health care, particularly patient care. Many nurses have earned a registered nurse degree, noted by RN in their title.

Nurse practitioner – A registered nurse with advanced training and emphasis in primary care.

Nutritionist – One who specializes in nutrition, meal planning and diet issues.

O

Occupational therapist – A health professional who teaches patients to reduce strain on joints while doing everyday activities; also known as an OT

Orthopaedic surgeon – A surgeon who specializes in diseases, injuries or problems of the bones

Orthopaedist – A physician who specializes in diseases, injuries or problems of the bones

Orthotic devices – Splints and braces that support and protect joints

Osteoarthritis – A disease causing cartilage breakdown in certain joints (spine, hands, hips, knees) resulting in pain and deformity

Osteolysis – Dissolution of bone, especially related to calcium loss in the bone

Osteophytes – Bony spurs that can develop on the ends of bones that can occur in osteoarthritis as a result of cartilage breakdown

Osteoporosis – A disease that causes bones to lose their mass, become porous and break easily

Osteotomy – A surgical procedure involving the cutting of bone, usually performed in cases of severe joint malalignment

GLOSSARY

P

Pain – A sensation or perception of hurting, ranging from discomfort to agony, that occurs in response to injury, disease or functional disorder. Pain is your body's alarm system, signaling that something is wrong. *Acute* pain is temporary and related to nerve endings stimulated by tissue damage and improves with healing. *Chronic* pain may be mild to severe but persists due to prolonged illness or damage.

Personal trainer – Person with expertise in directing fitness exercise programs.

Pharmacist – A professional licensed to prepare and dispense drugs.

Physiatrist – A physician who continues training after medical school and specializes in the field of physical medicine and rehabilitation.

Physical therapist – A health-care professional who has training and is licensed in the practice of physical therapy and may manage post-surgical rehabilitation exercises; also known as a PT.

Physical therapy – Methods and techniques of rehabilitation to restore function and prevent disability following surgery, injury or disease; may include applications of heat and cold, assistant devices, massage, and an individually tailored program of exercises.

Physician – A person who has successfully completed medical school and is licensed to practice medicine; also known as a doctor.

Physician, family – See *physician, primary care*.

Physician, general practitioner – See *physician, primary care*.

Physician, osteopathic – Doctors, also known as *osteopaths*, who base diagnosis and treatment on a philosophy that many illnesses are connected to disorders in the musculoskeletal system. Osteopaths have the same level of training as medical doctors, and may be primary care physicians or specialists, such as rheumatologists.

Physician, primary care – Physician to whom a family or individual goes initially when ill or for a periodic health check. This physician assumes medical coordination of care with other physicians for the patient with multiple health concerns.

Physician's assistant – A person trained, certified and licensed to assist physicians by recording medical history and performing the physical examination, diagnosis and treatment of commonly encountered medical problems under the supervision of a licensed physician.

Podiatrist – A health-care professional who specializes in care of the foot. Formerly called a chiropodist.

Press-fit – Style of adhering a joint component without cement.

Prostaglandin – A chemical in the body that influences inflammation and other processes.

Prosthesis – Artificial implant used to replace damaged or diseased body parts such as components of joints.

Psychiatrist – A physician who trains after medical school in the study, treatment and prevention of mental disorders. A psychiatrist may provide counseling and prescribe medicines and other therapies.

Psychologist – A trained professional, usually a PhD rather than an MD, who specializes in the mind and mental processes, especially in relation to human and animal behavior. A psychologist may measure mental abilities and provide counseling.

R

Range of motion (ROM) – The distance and angles at which your

GLOSSARY

joints can be moved, extended and rotated in various directions.

Reamer – Specially designed saw instrument used in joint surgery.

Relaxation – A state of release from mental or physical stress or tension.

Repetitive strain injury – Injury to the joints caused by repeated movements or strain to the joints, such as in work tasks or athletics.

Resection – Surgical procedure involving removing all or part of a bone.

Resection arthroplasty – A surgical procedure in which resection is done in conjunction with arthroplasty.

Revision – A surgical procedure to replace an artificial joint that was previously implanted but has been damaged or loosened.

Rheumatic disease – A general term referring to conditions characterized by pain and stiffness of the joints or muscles. The American College of Rheumatology currently recognizes over 100 rheumatic diseases. The term is often used interchangeably with "arthritis" (meaning joint inflammation), but not all rheumatic diseases affect the joints or involve inflammation.

Rheumatoid arthritis – A chronic, inflammatory autoimmune disease in which the body's protective immune system turns on the body and attacks the joints, causing pain, swelling and deformity.

Rheumatologist – A physician who pursues additional training after medical school and specializes in the diagnosis, treatment and prevention of arthritis and other rheumatic disorders.

S

Salicylates – A subcategory of NSAIDs, including aspirin, as well as topical creams that contain salicylic acid and relieve pain and inflammation.

ALL YOU NEED TO KNOW ABOUT JOINT SURGERY

Sam-e – Supplement purported to relieve pain and possibly ease depression symptoms; short for S-adenosylmethionine.

Self-management – The concept of a person having control of his or her disease and its management.

Skeletal muscles – The voluntary muscles that are primarily involved in moving parts of the body. "Voluntary" in this sense refers to muscles that move in response to our decisions to walk, bend, grasp and so on, as opposed to muscles such as the heart, which do their work without our willful direction.

Strain – Injury to a muscle, tendon or ligament by repetitive use, trauma or excessive stretching.

Strengthening exercises – Exercises that help maintain or increase muscle strength. See also *isometric exercises* and *isotonic exercises*.

Stress – The body's physical, mental and chemical reactions to frightening, exciting, dangerous or irritating circumstances.

Swedish massage – Traditional form of massage that involves kneading the muscles with applied pressure.

Synovectomy – Surgical removal of the synovium, or the lining of the joint.

Synovitis – Inflammation of the lining of the joint.

Synovium – The lining of the joint.

Synovial fluid – The fluid found in the joint.

T

TED hose – Support stockings worn just after surgery to prevent blood clots from developing in the legs.

GLOSSARY

Tendinitis – Inflammation of a tendon.

Tendon – A cord of dense, fibrous tissue uniting a muscle to a bone.

Tissue – A collection of similar cells that act together to perform a specific function in the body. The primary tissues are epithelial (skin), connective (ligaments and tendons), bone, muscle and nervous.

Trigger point therapy – See *neuro-muscular massage*.

Tumor – Mass of tissue or cellular growth that is independent of its surrounding structures in the body; can be benign (non-cancerous) or malignant (cancerous).

Unicondylar knee replacement – Less invasive form of knee replacement surgery in which damaged portions of a single condyle, cartilage and meniscus are removed, and bone is reshaped to fit a small implant.

USDA Food Guide Pyramid – A visual dietary guideline prepared by the United States Department of Agriculture. Stressing a diet rich in whole grains, lean proteins, fruits and vegetables, the diet is the current standard for nutrition in the United States.

Vertebrae – Joints of the spinal column.

Viscosupplementation – A treatment for knee osteoarthritis involving an injection of a hyaluronic acid product (viscosupplement) into the joint

Viscosupplements – Products injected to replace the hyaluronic acid missing from knee joints affected by osteoarthritis.

Vital signs – Term used to describe measurements of important physical indicators, such as body temperature, heart rate, blood pressure and others; these signs are monitored during and after surgery.

W

Warm-up – Gentle movement to warm up the muscles before performing stretches and more strenuous exercise.

X

X-ray – Diagnostic technique using electromagnetic radiation to obtain a two-dimensional image of bones and their structure.

Y

Yoga – Meaning "union," an ancient Indian practice that involves series of body postures called asanas. Yoga includes exercise, meditation and breathing components to improve posture and balance and help relieve stress on the joints, as well as emotional stress.

Resources for Good Living
WHAT THE ARTHRITIS FOUNDATION CAN DO FOR YOUR JOINT HEALTH

The Arthritis Foundation, the only national, voluntary health organization that works for the more than 43 million Americans with arthritis or related diseases, offers many valuable resources through more than 150 offices nationwide. The chapter that serves your area has information, products, classes and other services to help you take control of your arthritis or related condition. To find the chapter nearest you, call **800/283-7800** or search the Arthritis Foundation Web site at **www.arthritis.org**.

Programs and services

1. **Physician Referral** – Most Arthritis Foundation chapters can provide a list of doctors in your area who specialize in the evaluation and treatment of arthritis and arthritis-related diseases.

2. **Exercise Programs** – The Arthritis Foundation sponsors, develops and coordinates exercise programs for people with arthritis, featuring specially-trained instructors. They include:

   • **Walk With Ease** – This course allows participants to develop a walking plan that meets their individual needs, accompanied by the Arthritis Foundation book *Walk With Ease: Your Guide to Walking for Better Health, Improved Fitness and Less Pain.* A program leader's manual is also available for those interested in participating in a group format.

- **PACE** – (People with Arthritis Can Exercise): These courses feature gentle movements to increase joint flexibility, range of motion, stamina and muscle strength. An accompanying video is available for home use.
- **Arthritis Foundation Aquatic Program** – These water exercise programs, also held at many YMCAs, help relieve strain on muscles and joints. An accompanying PEP (Pool Exercise Program) video is available for home use.

3. **Self-Help Courses** – The Arthritis Foundation sponsors mutual-support groups that provide opportunities for discussion and problem-solving among people with arthritis. In addition, the Arthritis Foundation offers courses designed to help people actively manage their particular disease through exercise, medications, relaxation techniques, pain management, nutrition and more. These are the Fibromyalgia Self-Help Course and the Arthritis Self-Help Course.

Information and products

Find the latest information about arthritis, including research, medications, government advocacy, programs and services through one of the many information resources offered by the Arthritis Foundation:

1. **www.arthritis.org** – Information about arthritis is available 24 hours a day on the Internet at the Arthritis Foundation's interactive, comprehensive Web site. Find news about arthritis, ways to get involved,

and a variety of useful arthritis products, including books, brochures, videos and more. In addition, the Arthritis Foundation has a new interactive self-management guide for people with arthritis, **Connect and Control: Your Online Arthritis Action Guide**. Via questionnaire responses, *Connect and Control* helps participants create a customized management program for their unique situation.

2. **Arthritis Answers** – Call toll-free at 800/283-7800 for 24-hour, automated information about arthritis and Arthritis Foundation resources. Trained volunteers and staff are also available at your local Arthritis Foundation chapter to answer questions or refer you to physicians and other resources. For general questions about arthritis, you can also call 404-872-7100 ext. 1, or email questions to help@arthritis.org.

3. **Publications** – The Arthritis Foundation offers many publications to educate people with arthritis, as well as their families and friends, about diagnosis, medications, exercise, diet, pain management and more.

   - **Books** – The Arthritis Foundation publishes a variety of books on arthritis to help you learn to understand and manage your condition, live a healthier life, and cope with the emotional challenges that come with a chronic illness. Order books directly at www.arthritis.org or by calling 800/207-8633. All Arthritis Foundation books are available at your local bookstore.

- **Brochures:** The Arthritis Foundation offers brochures containing concise, understandable information on the many arthritis-related diseases and conditions. Topics include surgery, the latest medications, guidance for working with your doctors and self-managing your illness. Single copies are available free of charge at www.arthritis.org or by calling 800/283-7800.

- *Arthritis Today* – This award-winning bimonthly magazine provides the latest information on research, new treatments, trends and tips from experts and readers to help you manage arthritis. A one-year subscription to *Arthritis Today* is included when you become a member of the Arthritis Foundation. Annual membership is $20 and helps fund research to find cures for arthritis. Call 800/933-0032 for information.

- *Kids Get Arthritis Too* – This newsletter focusing on juvenile rheumatic diseases is published six times a year. Features speak to children and teens with the illness as well as to their parents. Stories examine the latest news in diagnosis, treatment and research of children's rheumatic diseases, as well as helpful ways kids can cope with their illnesses and the challenges they bring. This newsletter is now a benefit of membership in the Arthritis Foundation for people affected by juvenile rheumatic diseases. For information, call 800/283-7800.

Discussion Questions

Here are some items for discussion with members of your support group,
or for use on your own as food for thought.

- Why did you decide to explore surgery? When did you decide?
- What therapies, other than surgery, have you tried for your arthritis
  or joint pain? What has worked? What has not worked?
- What do you expect from your joint surgery? In the short term?
  In the long term?
- What activities do you hope to resume as a result of your
  joint surgery?
- What concerns do you have about surgery?
- Do you feel that your doctor has explained everything to you?
- What things would you most like to discuss with him?
- What are your concerns about rehabilitation or recovery?
  Discuss ways to alleviate these fears or solve the problems
  associated with recovery.
- What do you expect of your family members or loved ones
  during surgery and recovery? Discuss ways to communicate
  better with your loved ones to get the help you need.

A

Acetabulum, 153–154, 208
Acetaminophen, 41, 208
  joint surgery and, 91
Acetaminophen with codeine, 42
Activities
  resuming normal, 180–184
  weight loss and, 139–140
Acupressure, 208
Acupuncture, 49–50, 208
Acute illness, 208
Acute pain. *See* Pain
Aerobic, 208
Age, joint surgery and, 13–14, 16
Airport security, 199
Alcohol, 41, 45, 134, 135, 201
All You Need to Know
  About Back Pain, 27
Alternative therapy, 47, 48–51, 208
  acupuncture as, 49–50
  chiropractic as, 50
  evaluating, 52–53
  herbs and supplements as,
    51, 54–58, 92–93, 121
  hot and cold treatments as,
    42, 43, 58, 59, 60, 172
  joint surgery and, 92–93
  massage as, 61, 63
  vitamins as, 51–51
  water therapy as, 60–61
Ambien, 162
American Academy of
  Orthopaedic Surgeons, 110, 111
American Academy of Physical
  Medicine and Rehabilitation, 111
American College of
  Rheumatology (ACR), 41, 43, 208
American Dietetic Association, 201
American Lung Association, 201
American Physical
  Therapy Association, 111

Analgesics, 41–42, 160–161, 209
  topical, 42–43
Anesthesia, 12, 123, 152–153,
    159, 209
  epidural, 115, 152, 161, 214
  general, 35, 115–116, 158, 160
  local, 35
  regional, 114–115, 116, 160
  spinal, 115, 152
Anesthesiologists, 35, 152, 158, 209
Ankles, arthrodesis for, 77
Ankylosing spondylitis, 27, 50
Antibiotics, 93, 161, 167, 178, 209
Antioxidants, 50–51, 135, 209.
    See also Free radicals
ArthriCare, 42
Arthritis, 4–5, 209
  effect of, on joints, 28–29
  joint surgery and, 14–15
  types of, 25–27
Arthritis Foundation, xxi, 110, 111
  aquatics program, 60, 185, 205
  exercise programs, 204–205
  information and products
    from, 205–207
  physician referral by, 204
  self-help courses, 205
The Arthritis Foundation's Guide
  to Alternative Therapies, 49
Arthritis Foundation YMCA Aquatics
  Program (AFYAP), 60, 185
Arthritis Today, 207
Arthrodesis, 157, 209
  defined, 77
  joints used for, 77
  procedure in, 77
Arthroplasty, 209.
    See also Total joint replacement
Arthroscope, 78, 159
  in arthroscopy, 78
  in synovectomy, 81

Arthroscopy, 7, 11, 95,
    156–157, 192–193, 209
  defined, 78
  hospital stay for, 117
  joints used for, 78
  knee, 17, 78, 160
  for osteoarthritis, 26
  procedure in, 78–79
  recuperation from, 94
  regaining use of joint after, 191
Artificial joints, 29, 73, 74–75
Aspercreme, 43
Aspiration, 209
Aspirin (*Anacin, Ascriptin,*
    Bayer, Bufferin, Excedrin), 43
  glucosamine and, 56
  joint surgery and, 90
Assistive devices, 123, 126,
    164–165, 174, 176
ASU, 56, 210
Autoimmune disease, 26, 29, 210
Autologous blood transfusion,
    121, 210
Avocado oil, 56

B

Back kick, 145, 187
Back pain, 27
Ball-and-socket joints, 22, 210
Bathing, 174, 182
BenGay, 43
Beta carotene, 135
Bicycling, 144
Biologic response modifiers, 40, 210
Blood donation, 121
Blood-thinning medications
  glucosamine and, 56
  joint surgery and, 90
Board certification, 112
Body mechanics, 210

Bone and Joint Decade, 111
Bone cement, 75, 154, 155
Bone fusion, 77
    See also Arthrodesis
Bone loss, 193
Bone saw, 153, 159
Bone spurs, 28–29, 210
Bone tumor, 32
Boron, 56, 210
Boswellia, 57, 210
Braces, 47–48
Bunion, 80, 211
Bursae, 23, 211
Bursitis, 211

C

Calf stretch, 147
Calorie burning chart, 140
Camphor, 42
Cane, 172
Capsaicin, 42–43, 211
Capzasin-P, 43
Cardiac stress test, 86, 87
Cardiogram, 123
Cardiologist, 87
Cardiovascular exercise, 144
Cars, getting in and out of, 175–176
Cartilage, 23, 25, 28, 211
    breakdown of, 28
Catheter, 211
  in anesthesia, 115, 152–153
  urinary, 159, 161
Cefazolin, 161
Celecoxib (*Celebrex*), 45
  joint surgery and, 90
Cell saver, 121
Cemented/cementless implant,
    75–77, 154, 155, 211
Centers for Disease Control
    and Prevention, 111

Social workers, 37
Sock aid, 164–165, 174
Soybean oil, 56
Spinal anesthesia, 115, 152
Splints, 47–48
Sports, as cause of joint injuries, 30, 195
Sportscreme, 43
Steroids, 46
Stomach problems, 45
   risk factors for, 44
Strain, 222
Strengthening exercises, 145–148, 222
Stress, 222
Stress reduction, 201–202
Supplements, 51, 54–58
   joint surgery and, 92–93
   shopping for, 57
   substitutions for, 121
Surgeons, 158
   choosing, 64, 109–112
   orthopaedic, 33, 34, 64, 218
   podiatric, 35
   questions to ask potential, 112–113
Surgery. *See* Joint replacement surgery
Surgical team, 113–114
Swedish massage, 61, 222
Synovectomy, 27, 192–193, 222
   defined, 80–81
   joints used for, 81
   procedures in, 81
Synovial fluid, 23, 222
Synovitis, 222
Synovium, 23, 24, 80, 222

T

Tai chi, 185
TED hose, 163, 222
Telecommuting, 94
Tendinitis, 223
Tendons, 23, 223
Therapeutic Mineral Ice, 42

Thigh firmer and knee stretch, 146
Tibia, 154, 157
Tips for Good Living with
   Arthritis, 31, 126
Tissue, 223
Toe joint replacement, 155–156
Topical analgesics, 42–43
Total hip replacement, time for, 160
Total joint replacement, xx, 7, 16–17, 26
   for ankylosing spondylitis, 27
   cemented vs. cementless
     implants, 75–77
   defined, 73
   joints used for, 73
   procedure in, 73–74
   for rheumatoid arthritis, 27
   types of replacement parts, 74–75
Tramadol (*Ultram*), 42
Treatment, communication as
   key to successful, 37–39
Trigger point therapy, 61, 223
Tumors, 32, 223

U

Ulcers, 45, 51
   risk factors for, 44
Unicondylar knee replacement,
   156, 223
Ultram, 42
Urinary problems, as joint
   surgery risk factor, 88
USDA Food Guide Pyramid,
   134, 136, 223

V

Valdecoxib (*Bextra*), 45
   joint surgery and, 90
Vasculitis, 59
Vertebrae, 27, 223
Vicodin, 161

Viscosupplementation, 223
Viscosupplements, 47, 223
Vital signs, 159, 224
Vitamin C, 51, 135
Vitamin D, 51
Vitamin E, 135
Vitamins, 50–51

W

Walkers, 122, 126, 163, 164, 172, 175
Walking, 143–144, 200
Walk with Ease: Your Guide to Walking
    for Better Health, Improved Fitness
        and Less Pain, 144, 200, 204
Warfarin (*Coumadin*), 167
    joint surgery and, 90
Warm-up, 224
Water, 134, 136
Water exercise, 185
Water Exercise:
    Pools, Spas and Arthritis, 60
Water therapy, 60–61
Weight loss
    bicycling and, 144
    controlling portion sizes in, 138–139
    diet and, 50–51, 134–136
    exercise and, 139–140
Food Guide Pyramid and, 136
    health-care professionals in, 148–149
    maintaining, 187–188
    in preparing for surgery, 117–118
    reading food labels, 137–138
    tips for, before surgery, 132–140
    walking and, 143–144
Wheelchair, 164
Work
    as cause of joint injuries, 30
    recuperation time, 94–95
    returning to, 183–184
Wound care, 164

X

X-rays, 39, 123, 151, 224

Y

Yoga, 185, 224

Z

Zostrix, 43
Zostrix HP, 43

What's Wrong With My Back?

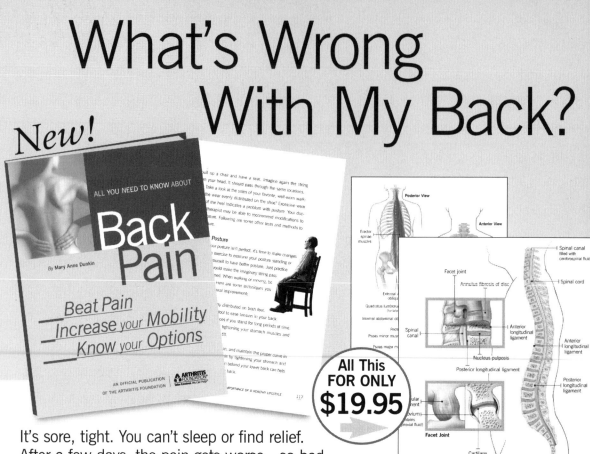

New!

ALL YOU NEED TO KNOW ABOUT

Back Pain

By Mary Anne Dunkin

Beat Pain
Increase your Mobility
Know your Options

AN OFFICIAL PUBLICATION OF THE ARTHRITIS FOUNDATION | ARTHRITIS FOUNDATION Take Control. We Can Help!

All This FOR ONLY $19.95

It's sore, tight. You can't sleep or find relief. After a few days, the pain gets worse…so bad that you have to miss a day of work. **What's wrong?**

You're experiencing **BACK PAIN**, one of the most common health problems in America today. For people of all ages, back pain is serious pain – and it requires serious attention from you and your doctor.

But what can you do about your back pain?

Now more than ever, there's a great deal you and your doctor can do to fight your back pain. Get all the latest treatments, techniques and prevention tips in a brand-new book from the Arthritis Foundation, *All You Need To Know About Back Pain: Beat Pain, Increase Your Mobility, Know Your Options*.

Are you ready to tell back pain to "back off"?
Order *All You Need To Know About Back Pain* today and find out how!

Get the facts on:

- The latest powerful drugs for your back

- Easy lifestyle changes to help you prevent back problems

- The truth about back surgery

- Alternative therapies that may really work for you

- New techniques to conquer your pain without pills

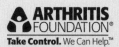